Certified Nurse Educator Review Book

The Official NLN Guide to the CNE® Exam

Second Edition

Certified Nurse Educator Review Book

The Official NLN Guide to the CNE® Exam

Second Edition

Edited by

Linda Caputi, EdD, MSN, RN, CNE, ANEF

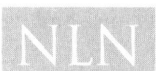

National League
for **Nursing**

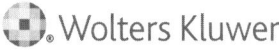

Philadelphia • Baltimore • New York • London
Buenos Aires • Hong Kong • Sydney • Tokyo

Vice President and Publisher: Julie K. Stegman
Director of Nursing Content Publishing: Renee Gagliardi
Director of Product Development: Jennifer K. Forestieri
Senior Development Editor: Meredith L. Brittain
Marketing Manager: Brittany Clements
Editorial Assistant: Molly Kennedy
Design Coordinator: Terry Mallon
Production Project Manager: Sadie Buckallew
Manufacturing Coordinator: Karin Duffield
Prepress Vendor: Aptara, Inc.

Caputi, L. (2020). *Certified Nurse Educator Review Book: The Official NLN Guide to the CNE® Exam.* Washington, DC: National League for Nursing.

9 8 7 6 5 4 3 2

Printed in USA

Library of Congress Cataloging-in-Publication Data

ISBN-13: 978-1-97515-405-9
Library of Congress Control Number: 2019917067
Cataloging in Publication data available on request from publisher.

DRC0620

About the Editor

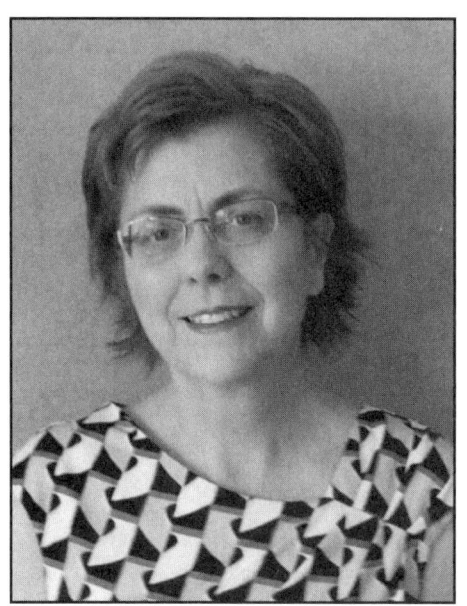

Linda Caputi, EdD, MSN, RN, CNE, ANEF is Professor Emeritus, College of DuPage. She has taught in LPN, ADN, BSN, and MSN programs. She is President of Linda Caputi, Inc., a nursing education consulting company. Dr. Caputi has consulted with hundreds of schools for over 30 years on topics related to revising curricula, teaching students to think, developing a concept-based curriculum, transforming clinical education, test item writing and analysis, using an evidence-based model for NCLEX® success, and numerous other nursing education topics. She has also presented at hundreds of workshops and nursing education conferences. She has published journal articles, educational software programs, and books, the most recent the student textbook *Think Like a Nurse: A Handbook*. Dr. Caputi is the editor of the column "Innovation Center" in the NLN's journal *Nursing Education Perspectives*. Dr. Caputi is a certified nurse educator, was inducted as a fellow into the NLN's Academy of Nursing Education, has served on the NLN's Board of Governors, and is a site visitor for the NLN's Commission for Nursing Education Accreditation.

About the Contributors

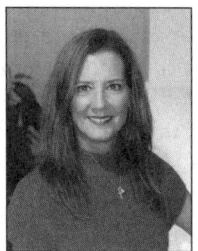

Donna Badowski, DNP, MSN, RN, CNE has been an assistant professor and assistant director of the RN to MS Program at the DePaul University School of Nursing (Chicago, Illinois) for the past four years. Prior to that, she was an associate professor and program chair at the College of DuPage nursing program (Glen Ellyn, Illinois). She completed research regarding simulation in nursing education related to facilitation strategies, use of electronic medical records in simulation, clinical simulation ratios, online asynchronous simulation, and synchronous telehealth simulation. She has held several committee positions with the International Association for Clinical Simulation and Learning (INACSL) and is currently the chair of the INACSL 2020 conference planning committee.

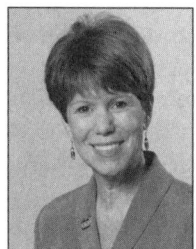

Gail Baumlein, PhD, MSN, RN, CNE, ANEF has been practicing nursing for almost 40 years, with 30 years in academia, having taught at all levels of nursing education. She has held faculty and leadership positions in schools, colleges, and universities and has been involved in the development of a multitude of new nursing programs and colleges. She is known for her presentations and writing in numerous areas, including using technology in education, active teaching strategies, best practices in online instruction, program accreditation, and assessment and evaluation. She is a certified nurse educator and a fellow in the NLN's Academy of Nursing Education. She has served on the NLN's Board of Governors and on the Board of Governors for the Ohio League for Nursing. She was honored as the University of Akron College of Nursing's distinguished alumni.

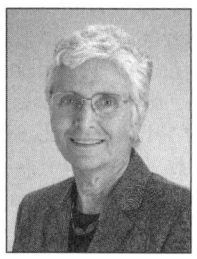

Wanda Blaser Bonnel, PhD, RN, APRN, ANEF serves as faculty member at University of Kansas, focusing on gerontological nursing, clinical education, and health professions educator roles. She is a fellow in the National League for Nursing's Academy of Nursing Education and has received multiple teaching awards. As a geriatric nurse practitioner, she serves on the *Journal of Gerontological Nursing* editorial board. She has had the leadership role in multiple funded grants, including the ongoing Health Professions Educator Certificate. Her funded research on best practices in faculty feedback to online students and observer role in simulation have yielded numerous national presentations and publications. Her two coauthored texts, *Teaching with Technologies in Nursing* and *Proposal Writing for Clinical Nursing and DNP Projects*, help prepare students for the changing world of health care. She enjoys her ongoing work with DNP and PhD student projects and dissertation research.

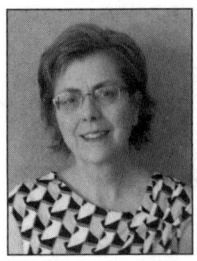

Linda Caputi, EdD, MSN, RN, CNE, ANEF is Professor Emeritus, College of DuPage. She has taught in LPN, ADN, BSN, and MSN programs. She is President of Linda Caputi, Inc., a nursing education consulting company. Dr. Caputi has consulted with hundreds of schools for over 30 years on topics related to revising curricula, teaching students to think, developing a concept-based curriculum, transforming clinical education, test item writing and analysis, using an evidence-based model for NCLEX® success, and numerous other nursing education topics. She has also presented at hundreds of workshops and nursing education conferences. She has published journal articles, educational software programs, and books, the most recent the student textbook *Think Like a Nurse: A Handbook*. Dr. Caputi is the editor of the column "Innovation Center" in the NLN's journal *Nursing Education Perspectives*. Dr. Caputi is a certified nurse educator, was inducted as a fellow into the NLN's Academy of Nursing Education, has served on the NLN's Board of Governors, and is a site visitor for the NLN's Commission for Nursing Education Accreditation.

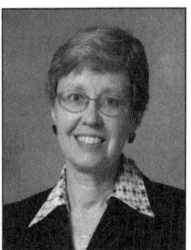

Marilyn Frenn, PhD, RN, CNE, FTOS, ANEF, FAAN is a professor at Marquette University College of Nursing. Her research currently involves measuring student response to interprofessional education programs. She has chaired several dissertations related to nursing education with vulnerable groups of students and conducted qualitative studies to understand teaching excellence from student and faculty perspectives. She contributed to the first edition of this book and to the new *NLN Core Competencies for Nurse Educators: A Decade of Influence*. She currently serves on the National League for Nursing (NLN) Commission for Nursing Education Accreditation Standards Committee and previously served on the NLN Board of Governors and Membership Committee, and as President of WI League for Nursing.

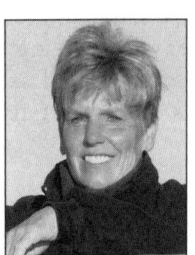

Susan Luparell, PhD, RN, CNE, ANEF is an associate professor in the College of Nursing at Montana State University, Bozeman, Montana, where she has been involved in both the baccalaureate and graduate nursing programs for 20 years. A fellow in the Academy of Nursing Education, Susan is an expert on the dynamics between teacher and learner in nursing education as well as a nationally recognized speaker and author on the topic of incivility in nursing education. Her scholarship focuses on the ethical implications of incivility in health care, including how it affects others and how it can be managed in academic as well as in clinical settings. Additionally, she has served multiple terms on the NLN's Research Review Panel and is a seasoned instructor who has received multiple commendations over the years for excellence in teaching.

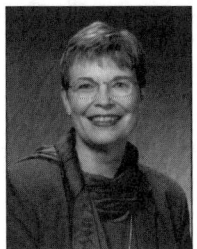

Nancy C. Sharts-Hopko, PhD, RN, CNE, ANEF, FAAN is a professor in the M. Louise Fitzpatrick College of Nursing at Villanova University, where she served for 13 years as the inaugural director of the PhD Program. Following graduation from Indiana University, she practiced in the area of neonatal intensive care. After studying nursing education at New York University, she has taught at the undergraduate and graduate levels for 41 years. Additionally, she has taught and consulted in universities in Japan and Bangladesh. Her research in the areas of women's health and nursing education has been published in numerous peer-reviewed journals. Dr. Sharts-Hopko serves as an accreditation site visitor for professional and regional organizations, and she served on the National League for Nursing's Commission on Nursing Education, which she chaired from 2009 to 2011.

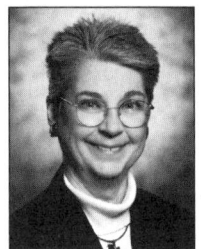

Theresa M. "Terry" Valiga, EdD, RN, CNE, FAAN, ANEF is Professor Emerita at Duke, Senior Visiting Professor at Virginia Commonwealth University, and Fellow in Villanova's PhD Program. Previous appointments include NLN's Chief Program Officer and faculty at Trenton State, Seton Hall, Georgetown, Villanova, and Fairfield, where she was the Dean of Nursing for four years. Dr. Valiga has received grants to study student learning, cognitive/intellectual development, curriculum design, leadership development, student perspectives of excellent teachers, and student evaluations of courses and teachers; published extensively, including five coauthored books on education and leadership, the latter now being prepared in its sixth edition; presented at national and international conferences; served as a consultant to many schools of nursing in and outside the United States; served on several national governing boards; and currently serves on the NLN's Commission for the Certified Nurse Educator program and as a faculty adviser for Sigma Theta Tau's Experienced Nurse Educator Leadership Academy. Dr. Valiga received Sigma's Elizabeth Russell Belford Founders Award for Excellence in Nursing Education and the NLN's Outstanding Leadership in Nursing Education Award, and she is a fellow in the Academy of Nursing Education and the American Academy of Nursing.

Foreword

Continually striving for excellence in nursing education and never settling for the status quo is an important distinction for all nurse educators. Becoming a certified nurse educator is one way to demonstrate such merit. It is a mark of professionalism and sends a message loud and clear to students, other nurse educators, practice partners, and interprofessional colleagues of your strong expertise in the specialty role of nurse educator.

There are more than 4,000 certified nurse educators nationally. You have the opportunity to take either the Certified Nurse Educator (CNE®) or the Certified Academic Clinical Nurse Educator (CNE®cl) examination. The National League for Nursing's Certified Nurse Educator (CNE) credential is the only official recognition for nurse educators to demonstrate their knowledge and expertise in academic nursing, including curricular design, teaching and learning, evaluation, and facilitating students' learning in the clinical area by connecting the dots between classroom and clinical.

Preparing for the nurse educator certification examination should not be taken lightly; luckily, there are great resources that can support your pursuit toward excellence. One of the best resources that I can recommend is the second edition of the *Certified Nurse Educator Review Book: The Official NLN Guide to the CNE® Exam*, edited by Dr. Linda Caputi. Each chapter continues to be based on the Core Competencies of the Academic Nurse Educator that are addressed in the *Certified Nurse Educator (CNE®) Handbook* and are a part of the CNE Test Plan. The chapter authors are literally a "Who's Who" in nursing education, delivering detailed descriptions of the competencies and relevant research followed by practice questions that test your knowledge of each chapter's content. In the second edition, scenarios have been added that address the nurse educator's practice.

In this review book, Dr. Linda Caputi, a CNE colleague I have had the pleasure of working with through the years, has captured the necessary components needed to be successful in taking the certification examination. She has a long-term association with the NLN as a past member of the Board of Governors and presently is a fellow in the Academy of Nursing Education. A prolific writer, nurse educator consultant to all types of nursing education programs, and innovation editor for the NLN's journal *Nursing Education Perspectives*, Dr. Caputi travels the country helping nurse educators and nursing programs deliver optimal innovative programming that produces nursing graduates who are prepared to provide quality, safe, team-based patient care.

As a dean, I strongly promote and encourage faculty to obtain their CNE certification. In fact, the College purchased a copy of the first edition of Dr. Caputi's review book for all faculty members because I felt it was such a valuable resource. The second edition is even better!

Marsha Howell Adams, PhD, RN, CNE, ANEF, FAAN
Dean and Professor
College of Nursing
The University of Alabama in Huntsville
Past President of the National League for Nursing (2013–2015)

Preface

Welcome to the second edition of the *Certified Nurse Educator Review Book: The Official NLN Guide to the CNE® Exam*! The National League for Nursing is delighted to present this resource for nurse educators. The purpose of this book is to provide an overall review in preparation for taking the CNE examination based on the CNE examination test blueprint. Therefore, this book is intended to supply the type of information that relates to each category on the test blueprint.

Book Organization

The book is divided into chapters—one chapter for each of the eight categories on the CNE test blueprint. Each chapter presents an overview of the content included on that exam blueprint.

Please note that the book does not represent an exhaustive discussion of all possible topics that may appear on the examination. As those who have taken a certification examination in nursing know, it would be difficult, if not impossible, to completely cover all possible information related to each of the areas of the CNE test blueprint. However, this book presents the major categories, then provides readers with concrete information to guide their study.

Each chapter contains practice test items that reflect those on the CNE exam. Rationales for correct and incorrect answers are included.

What is New to the Second Edition

The second edition of the *Certified Nurse Educator Review Book: The Official NLN Guide to the CNE® Exam* continues to offer sound guidance to those studying for the CNE examination. This edition features the following enhancements since the first edition:

- updated content
- additional bulleted lists and tables
- example scenarios that describe when faculty might apply some of the content in each chapter; this provides faculty with a realistic context for when the topic might be useful
- expanded number of practice questions
- rationales for all answer options for the practice questions

Studying for the Exam

A common question asked by attendees of a CNE review course is, "How should I study for the exam?" One approach is the following:

1. Review the CNE eligibility requirements (available online at www.nln.org).
2. Read the current CNE *Candidate Handbook* (available online at www.nln.org).
3. Set a target date for taking the CNE examination.

4. Review this book.
5. Develop a list of topics with which you are unfamiliar and/or consider areas in which you need further study.
6. Develop a calendar of study.
7. Consult the publications listed in the CNE *Candidate Handbook* and review the areas you identified as needing further study.
8. Take the NLN's self-assessment examination (SAE), which is available for purchase at http://www.nln.org/Certification-for-Nurse-Educators/cne/exam-prep/self-assessment-examination. The Internet-based SAE is half the length of the actual examination, offering valuable practice by taking CNE-type questions written by CNE item writers. Rationales for correct and incorrect answers are included.
9. Based on your results on the SAE, determine areas in which you may need additional study.
10. Review the identified areas for further study using this book as well as other publications listed in the CNE *Candidate Handbook*.
11. Optional: Attend a CNE review course. You can find information about CNE review courses on the NLN website or register for the CNE review course offered online by the NLN. Information is available on the NLN website at http://www.nln.org/professional-development-programs/nln-ondemand-courses.
12. Take the CNE examination.

It is helpful to determine your individual preferences for study. Whereas some candidates prefer to study alone, others find forming a study group with other faculty to be very helpful. A convenient way to form a group is to work with faculty within your own school. Groups can meet in the workplace over lunch or at another convenient time.

CNE Research

Since the initial offering of the CNE examination, studies have been conducted to better understand candidate performance as well as the perceived value of nurse educator certification. An analysis of first-time pass/fail performance on the CNE exam was initially conducted by Ortelli (2013; 2016). Lundeen (2014; 2018) then analyzed the performance of candidates who were unsuccessful on the CNE examination, while Christensen (2015) analyzed factors related to success on the CNE examination based on the revised eligibility criteria. The results of this research provide insights about the characteristics of nurse educators who achieved first-time success and those who need additional attempts. To understand the perceived value of certification, Barbé (2015) validated the Perceived Value of Certification Tool© with a focus on nurse educator certification (PVCT-NE). This tool was then used to conduct a national survey, which revealed that nurse educator certification is positively perceived by nursing faculty (Barbé & Kimble, 2017).

Certification as a Mark of Distinction

Taking the CNE examination is an exciting adventure. Certification is a mark of professionalism. Certification as a nurse educator is a mark of distinction for nursing faculty and recognition of the advanced specialty role of the academic nurse educator. Best wishes as you embark on this excellence initiative offered by the National League for Nursing.

Acknowledgments

I hereby acknowledge the many people who worked tirelessly for over a decade to make the CNE program a reality. As explained by Dr. Ortelli (2010), the NLN engaged in a series of tasks that culminated in the current CNE examination. These tasks resulted in the completion of:

- a think tank in 2001
- a position statement, Preparation of Nurse Educators, issued by the NLN Board of Governors in 2002
- a feasibility study/needs assessment in 2003, which revealed that 80 percent of deans and directors saw certification of nurse educators as beneficial to their programs
- the Core Competencies of Nurse Educators, developed by a task group on Nurse Educator Competencies
- a task analysis that provided content validity to the certification examination
- the CNE test blueprint
- the CNE examination

These tasks brought the test to nurse educators for the first time in September 2005. Since 2005, thousands of nurse educators have taken the examination and are certified. These early efforts built a strong foundation on which the NLN continues this important work.

I would like to thank all of the chapter authors. As the editor, I understand that the quality of this book is a direct expression of the work of the chapter authors. Each author represents nursing education at its very best; I am very grateful for the time and expertise they unselfishly shared to make this book a reality.

Finally, I am grateful for the time and work of Dr. Elaine Tagliareni, Dr. Barbara Patterson, and Amy McGuire of the National League for Nursing. These colleagues carry out the behind-the-scenes administrative work for much of what we enjoy from the NLN. I appreciate the patience and professionalism they provided during all of our interactions.

Linda Caputi, EdD, MSN, RN, CNE, ANEF
Editor

References

Barbé, T. (2015). Preliminary psychometric analysis of the modified perceived value of certification tool for the nurse educator. *Nursing Education Perspectives, 36*(4), 244–248. doi:10.5480/14-1429

Barbé, T. & Kimble, L. P. (2017). What is the value of nurse educator certification? A comparison study of certified and noncertified nurse educators. *Nursing Education Perspectives, 39*(2), 66–71. doi: 10.1097/01. NEP.0000000000000261

Christensen, L. S. (2015). *Factors related to success on the certified nurse educator (CNE®) examination.* Retrieved from ProQuest Dissertations & Theses Global. (1700787339)

Lundeen, J. D. (2014). *Analysis of unsuccessful candidate performance on the certified nurse educator examination.* Retrieved from ProQuest Dissertations & Theses Global. (1658786247)

Lundeen, J.D. (2018). Analysis of first-time unsuccessful attempts on the certified nurse educator examination. *Nursing Education Perspectives, 39*(2), 72–79. doi:10.1097/01.NEP.0000000000000276

Ortelli, T. (2010). The certified nurse educator credential. In L. Caputi (Ed.), *Teaching nursing: The art and science*, pp. 564–585. Glen Ellyn, IL: DuPage Press.

Ortelli, T. (2013). *Evaluating the knowledge of those who teach: An analysis of candidates' performance on the certified nurse educator (CNE) examination.* ProQuest Dissertations & Theses Global. (3617863)

Ortelli, T. A. (2016). Candidates' first-time performance on the Certified Nurse Educator examination. *Nursing Education Perspectives, 37*(4), 189–193. doi:10.1097/01.NEP.0000000000000024

Contents

Facilitate Learning

Donna Badowski, DNP, MSN, RN, CNE

The CNE® Test Plan lists the following for the area of Facilitate Learning:

Facilitate Learning

A. Implement a variety of teaching strategies appropriate to:
   1. content
   2. setting (i.e., clinical vs. classroom)
   3. learner needs
   4. learning style
   5. desired learner outcomes
   6. method of delivery (e.g., face-to-face, remote, simulation)

B. Use teaching strategies based on:
   1. educational theory
   2. evidence-based practices related to education

C. Modify teaching strategies and learning experiences based on consideration of learners':
   1. cultural background
   2. past clinical experiences
   3. past educational and life experiences
   4. generational groups (i.e., age)

D. Use information technologies to support the teaching-learning process.

E. Practice skilled oral and written (including electronic) communication that reflects an awareness of self and relationships with learners (e.g., evaluation, mentorship, and supervision).

F. Communicate effectively orally and in writing with an ability to convey ideas in a variety of contexts.

G. Model reflective thinking practices, including critical thinking

H. Create opportunities for learners to develop their own critical thinking skills.

I. Create a positive learning environment that fosters a free exchange of ideas.

J. Show enthusiasm for teaching, learning, and the nursing profession that inspires and motivates students.

K. Demonstrate personal attributes that facilitate learning (e.g., caring, confidence, patience, integrity, respect, and flexibility).

L. Respond effectively to unexpected events that affect instruction.

M. Develop collegial working relationships with clinical agency personnel to promote positive learning environments.

N. Use knowledge of evidence-based practice to instruct learners.

O. Demonstrate ability to teach clinical skills.

P. Act as a role model in practice settings.

Q. Foster a safe learning environment.

INTRODUCTION

One of the primary competencies of the Academic Nurse Educator (ANE) is to effectively facilitate learning. This is validated by the fact that this competency is the largest content area on the National League for Nursing (NLN) Certified Nurse Educator (CNE®) exam (NLN, 2018a). Within this core competency, the NLN has delineated required roles that facilitate learning to achieve the desired cognitive, affective, and psychomotor outcomes required of entry-level nursing students. This chapter focuses on each of these roles within the competency of Facilitate Learning.

IMPLEMENT A VARIETY OF TEACHING STRATEGIES

There are multiple variables to consider before implementing a teaching strategy. Effective ANEs consider the content, setting, learner needs, learning style, desired learner outcomes, and method of delivery to create optimal learning conditions (NLN, 2018a). Figure 1.1 shows the relationship of these variables when selecting the appropriate teaching strategy. This requires multiple types of approaches to facilitate learning in a variety of contexts to meet learner needs and achieve desired outcomes.

Content

The first variable affecting teaching strategies is content. ANEs consider what is being taught before deciding on a teaching strategy to meet learning outcomes. The focus on this variable is not deciding on the specific content to teach but rather how to best facilitate the learning of previously chosen content from curriculum

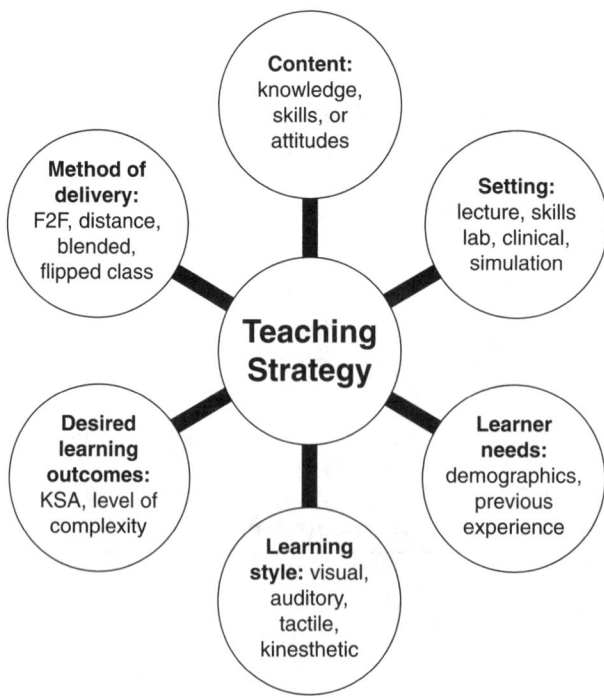

FIGURE 1.1 Variables in implementing teaching strategies.

development. Content is derived from the curriculum, the focus of another core competency, to be reviewed in a later chapter. The ANE considers whether the content requires acquisition of knowledge, a skill, or an attitude. A strategy designed to facilitate learning in the cognitive domain most likely will not be an appropriate strategy to facilitate learning in the psychomotor or affective domains.

Setting

Next, the ANE considers in which learning environment the content will be covered. Nursing students learn in a variety of settings; each setting requires different teaching strategies to meet learning outcomes. The classroom setting is the traditional environment for presenting information. Here, faculty deliver information and create active learning strategies for students. In contrast, the skills and simulation laboratories, and clinical environments, are ripe for action-oriented learning centered on students practicing skills and critical thinking. Regardless of the setting, all learning should be student centered with active engagement by students in the learning process (Benner, Sutphen, Leonard, & Day, 2010; NLN, 2006).

Learner Needs

ANEs also consider the students' gaps in knowledge, which is the gap between what learners know and what they need to know (Kitchie, 2019). Nursing students enter nursing programs with their individual set of prerequisite knowledge, skills, and attitudes related to health care and nursing based on their individual life experiences/education. Therefore, students present to the program with their own individual gaps in knowledge, creating a multitude of learner needs. Furthermore, veteran status and potential presence of learning disabilities bring even more diverse learner needs to the learning environment (Popkess & Frey, 2016). It is best to use a variety of teaching strategies with a student-centered approach to meet these varied learner needs. The ANE cannot use a "one-size-fits-all" approach when implementing teaching strategies. When learning environments are tailored to student needs, improved outcomes are achieved and course failures are minimized (Popkess & Frey, 2016).

Learning Style

Learning styles are the methods by which a student perceives and processes information (Kitchie, 2019). Kitchie (2019) presents a variety of learning style models. However, this section will present only the Dunn and Dunn Learning Styles Model. It identifies five stimuli that affect learning: environmental, emotional, sociological, physical, and psychological. With these stimuli in mind, ANEs need to consider the following questions regarding learners before choosing teaching strategies:

- What type of sounds, temperatures, lighting, and environmental designs are preferred by my students?
- How much motivation do my students prefer?
- Are my students self-directed and assume responsibility?
- Do my students prefer structure?
- Do my students prefer learning in solitude, through teamwork, or with teacher guidance?

Table 1.1

Learning Styles Tailored to Teaching Strategies

Learning Style	Teaching Strategies
Visual	Concept map, observing a skill, reading PowerPoint slides
Auditory	Lecture, podcasting lecture; group discussion
Tactile	Typing and posting to a class wiki or discussion board
Kinesthetic	Role play, simulation

- What are the perceptual (auditory, visual, tactile, kinesthetic) preferences of my students?
- Do my students learn better when they are drinking fluids or chewing food/gum?
- During what time of day do my students prefer to learn?
- Do my students prefer to move about or sit still?
- Do my students prefer conceptual models or more sequential models?
- Do my students prefer to participate verbally in groups or are they more reflective?

Tailoring activities so that students' natural dominant traits for learning can be used will allow them to learn better (Rundle & Dunn, 2008). Table 1.1 provides examples of teaching strategies tailored to specific learning styles.

Desired Learner Outcomes

The starting point for any teaching plan is the learner outcomes. ANEs consider the end product of the learning process before selecting a teaching strategy. Learner outcomes drive the teaching strategy by:

- articulating what students should know (knowledge), be able to do (skills), or value (attitude)
- expressing the level of complexity of the learning through action verbs using Bloom's taxonomy in the outcome statement (Oermann & Gaberson, 2017)

To effectively facilitate learning, ANEs directly align teaching strategies to the student learning outcomes, which are clearly stated in the course syllabus. When teaching strategies do not align with learning outcomes, students are at risk for not achieving the intended learning. This is analogous to packing for a vacation— if the traveler does not pack with the destination in mind, there is a risk that the clothes packed will not align with the weather patterns of the destination point.

Method of Delivery

The method in which learning is delivered is the final variable impacting teaching strategies. There are multiple ways in which learning is delivered in nursing programs:

- Face-to-face education is exactly what the name infers. The learning occurs with the ANE and students in the same location at the same time.

- Distance education requires the ANE to facilitate learning in a location other than that of the students. It can occur online or through videoconferencing. Online delivery is accomplished with a Learning Management System (LMS) and can further be delivered in two ways:
  - asynchronously—faculty and students log into the LMS independent of each other
  - synchronously—faculty and students are together in the LMS in real time (McAfooes, 2016)
- Blended learning is a combination of both face-to-face and distance education methods (McAfooes, 2016).
- Flipped classroom is a method in which direct instruction occurs outside the class-room, as preclass activities, so that class time can be spent engaging the learners in active strategies to promote higher levels of thinking (Caputi & Frank, 2019).
- Simulation is the creation of a particular set of conditions resembling authentic situations possible in real life (INACSL Standards Committee, 2016). Faculty design simulation-based experiences that allow participants to develop or enhance knowledge, skills, and/or attitudes and provide students with the opportunity to analyze and respond to realistic clinical situations (INACSL Standards Committee, 2016).
- Service learning is a method of education in which students participate in service to a community. It is a reciprocal learning experience whereby the service provided by the students meets the needs of the community being served as well as the student learning outcomes (Mueller, 2016). This method is intended to promote civic engagement, cultural competency, and critical thinking (Rodriguez & Lapiz-Bluhm, 2018).

Research shows that students value the face-to-face method for the realism, immediacy of feedback, and human connectedness that it offers (Gruendemann, 2011). However, it is not necessarily the preferred context in which to learn. Wells and Dellinger (2011) examined three methods of delivery; face-to-face, online, and use of compressed video for students to attend classes in a different location from the host site. They found that it was not so much the method of delivery but rather the quality of instruction that mattered. Additionally, there was no difference in perceived learning, feelings of connectedness, and interactions between student-student and student-instructor interactions. Therefore, it is important to create strategies that not

---

Scenario 1.1

An ANE is teaching the didactic portion of advanced medical-surgical nursing. One of the course learning outcomes is "Apply the nursing process when caring for patients requiring advanced nursing concepts and skills." Congestive heart failure (CHF) is the exemplar for the concept of perfusion. The ANE plans to deliver a 15-minute lecture with PowerPoint slides and then have students form small groups to work on a case study of a patient with CHF. They will create a concept map of the care for that patient during the group work.

Consider:
1. Has this ANE taken into account all of the variables discussed that impact implementation of teaching strategies?
2. How can the number of different activities facilitate learning for these students?
3. Will these strategies allow the learners to meet the lesson objectives?
4. How do these strategies address the learning styles of the students?
5. How do these strategies take into account the learning needs of the students?

only facilitate achievement of learning of outcomes but also promote student-student and student-instructor connections in all methods.

EVIDENCE-BASED TEACHING STRATEGIES

Educational Theory

Learning is a complex process that results in a permanent change in "mental processing, emotional functioning, skill, and/or behavior as a result of exposure to different experiences" (Braungart, Braungart, & Gramet, 2019, p. 70). Learning theories explain the relationships among the concepts present in the learning process (Candela, 2016). They provide the foundation for creating innovative teaching strategies to facilitate student learning.

ANEs use learning theories to guide the selection of teaching strategies, which need to align not only with faculty preferences but also with the nursing program's philosophy and be able to meet learning outcomes. Table 1.2 contains a list of some common learning theories, categorized by their paradigm, a brief description, and example implications for ANEs (Candela, 2016).

Table 1.2

Learning Theories and ANE Example Implications

Theory	Description	Example ANE Implications
Behaviorism	Learning is focused on consequences and reinforcements.	Observable and measurable behavioral objectives and learning outcomes Learning experiences allowing for positive reinforcement with ongoing feedback
Cognitivism	Learning is focused on mental processes and modifying cognitive structures to form new mental models.	Active learning strategies that teach students how to think and discover new meaning
Constructivist • Social Learning Theory • Sociocultural Learning • Situated Cognition	Learner constructs new knowledge from existing knowledge. Learning through observation of others Learning through interaction with the "expert," with "expert" eventually withdrawing support as student demonstrates mastery Learning occurs in the context of real-world experience (actual nursing practice)	Group interactions Communication and collaboration with other students Simulation Reflection of clinical practice experiences in post conference Debriefing after simulation Role modeling Role-play
Cognitive Development Theories • Adult Learning Theory • Novice-to-Expert	Learning through sequential development over time with a focus of information processing emphasizing understanding and acquisition of new knowledge Learners are self-directed and use past experiences in the learning process Learning occurs through levels of knowledge and experience throughout the nursing program	Active learning strategies in which students discover meaning Information processing strategies Reflection of new learning with past experiences Modifications to teaching based on continued assessments of performance Used as a guide for capstone projects

Evidence-Based Teaching Practices

Just as clinical nurses use evidence to inform nursing care provided to patients, ANEs use evidence to inform teaching and learning practices provided to nursing students (NLN, 2016a). Evidence-based teaching practice is the use of evidence to inform ANEs on how best to facilitate learning so that learning outcomes can be met (Kalb, O'Conner-Von, Brockway, Rierson, & Sendelbach, 2015). Evidence includes research, professional judgment and expertise, and student preferences and values. ANEs provide a variety of evidence-based teaching strategies to meet multiple learner needs and student learning styles (Breytenbach, Ham-Baloyi, & Jordan, 2017). Some examples of evidence-based, student-centered teaching strategies follow:

- Flipped classroom (Betihavas, Bridgman, Kornhaber, & Cross, 2016; Caputi & Frank, 2019; Njie-Carr et al., 2017)
  - Preclass, self-directed individual activities frequently occur online via module assignments.
  - In-class group activities focus on empowering students to apply preclass assignments, allowing integration of collaboration, active learning, and team-based learning.
  - Benefits: improved active engagement, performance/academic outcomes, course satisfaction, clinical outcomes through increased self-confidence and patient interactions.
  - Weaknesses: student concerns regarding increased amount of work; students' perception of being at a distance from faculty.
- Active learning strategies (Caputi & Frank, 2019)
  - Learner-centered approaches to facilitate learning.
  - Allow for integration of new knowledge aligning with constructivist learning theory.
  - Problem solving, inquiry-based learning.
  - Students prefer active learning strategies over traditional once they are exposed to them.
- Games (Aljezawi & Albashtawy, 2015; Breytenbach et al., 2017)
  - Improve retention of knowledge content and enhance student satisfaction.
  - Can be used to assess knowledge at the beginning of class or assess understanding at the end of class.
- Collaborative testing (Wiggs, 2010)
  - Students collaborate in small groups for test taking.
  - Benefits: allows for critical thinking and team-based learning
  - Weaknesses: peer pressure from having to be prepared to defend answers.
- Response systems (Efstathiou & Bailey, 2012; Mareno, Bremner, & Emerson, 2010; Revell & McCurry, 2010)
  - Use a personal response system (PRS) to engage the learner in class by polling students on questions for immediate feedback as the system displays class poll results.
  - Engage higher-level thinking and decision-making, facilitate teacher-student communication, and help faculty gauge student understanding.
- Simulation-based experiences (Hayden, Smiley, Alexander, Kardong-Edgren, & Jeffries, 2014)
  - Activities that represent actual or potential clinical situations allowing learners to develop knowledge, skills, and/or attitudes.
  - Provide opportunities for analyzing and responding to realistic situations (INACSL Standards Committee, 2016).

Scenario 1.2

An ANE who is facilitating a simulated learning experience places the student observers directly in the simulated patient room. The observers are instructed to watch for compromises to patient safety. If a compromise is discovered, the observers are able to provide support to the students who are actively engaged in the simulated learning experience. Furthermore, the role of the nurse in the simulated learning experience may seek support from the observers when unsure how to proceed safely.

Consider:
1. What are your thoughts on the student observer role potentially becoming an active participant in the simulation?
2. Will this strategy be a barrier to facilitating learning for the role of the observer, the role of the nurse, or both?
3. Is there a theory that supports the use of this strategy?
4. What would be your plan for the observer roles to facilitate learning and what theory would guide your decision?

MODIFY TEACHING STRATEGIES AND LEARNING EXPERIENCES BASED ON CONSIDERATION OF LEARNERS' CHARACTERISTICS

Although limited, student diversity exists in nursing programs. Percentages of minorities enrolled in basic registered nursing programs in 2016 were Black 10.8 percent, Hispanic 8.1 percent, Asian/Pacific Islander 5.5 percent, American Indian 0.7 percent, and other/unknown 4.5 percent (NLN, 2016b). The percentage of men enrolled in practical/vocational to doctorate programs is near 15 percent (NLN, 2016c). Diversity related to age is another variable impacting the way students learn. There are a variety of generations enrolled across all nursing programs (NLN, 2016d). ANEs modify teaching strategies to meet the needs of the diverse student population to retain and graduate students who will match the diversity of patients (Institute of Medicine [IOM], 2011). ANEs need to ensure inclusive environments that accommodate the diverse students in nursing education (Alexander, 2016). Table 1.3 offers recommendations for creating inclusivity and addressing diversity. The combination of age, gender, race/ethnicity, and life experiences in the class can facilitate learning by exposing students to rich, diverse perspectives that contribute to advancing the nursing profession and providing better care to patients (IOM, 2011).

USE INFORMATION TECHNOLOGIES TO SUPPORT THE TEACHING-LEARNING PROCESS

The NLN calls for nursing education to "teach with and about technology" (NLN, 2015, p. 4) to improve health care interventions and outcomes. ANEs intentionally incorporate technologies in support of the teaching-learning process to better prepare the nursing workforce. Digital technology connects students, faculty experts, patients, and virtual clinical experiences in interactive ways to facilitate learning (Thompson, 2016). Table 1.4 offers ways to integrate technology in the classroom, clinical, skills and simulation laboratories, and online learning environments.

Table 1.3

Diversity and Example Strategies for Inclusivity

Diversity	Strategies for Inclusivity
Cultural background (race/ethnicity, gender, sexual orientation)	Create inclusive learning environments requiring mutual respect and encouraging sharing of multiple perspectives. Apply gender-neutral language unless gender affects the objectives. Provide time for responses to Socratic questioning, allowing time for English language learners to translate their thoughts. Ask students to write a question each week pertaining to the lesson and then read the question to the class (Alexander, 2016).
Past clinical experiences	Allow students to share prior clinical experiences in discussion topics for deeper learning experiences (Knowles, 1980; Ramsden, 2013).
Past educational and life experiences	Allow students to share prior learning and personal life experiences into discussion topics for deeper learning experiences (Knowles, 1980; Ramsden, 2013).
Generational groups (i.e., age)	Incorporate active learning, group activities, and technology to meet the preferences of Generation Y (millennials) born between 1970 and 1990 along with Generation Z born after 1990, which are the largest demographic population in nursing programs (NLN, 2016d; Popkess & Frey, 2016). Incorporate occasional teacher-centered lecture to appeal to older generations (Popkess & Frey, 2016).

Table 1.4

Use of Technology

Setting	Technology to Support the Teaching-Learning Process
Classroom (Badowski, Horsley, Rossler, Mariani, & Gonzalez, 2018; Thompson, 2016)	Smartboards with visual displays throughout the room for easy accessibility and visualization for group work Teleconferences, telehealth, point-to-point conferences Internet for accessing literature, news, videos Allow student use of mobile devices for student access to Internet, e-books, and nursing software applications, such as drug guides or health-related applications. Personal response systems Simulated electronic health record
Clinical (Thompson, 2016)	Mobile devices for drug guides, clinical calculators, medical dictionary, literature searches—however, policies must be in place to ensure proper use
Skills laboratory (Badowski et al., 2018; Jarvill, Kelly, & Krebs, 2018; Staykova, Von Stewart, & Staykov, 2017)	Video simulations Expert role modeling videos Simulated electronic health record
Simulation laboratory (Badowski et al., 2018; Thompson, 2016)	Telehealth simulation Mobile devices for drug guides, clinical calculators, medical dictionary, literature searches—however, policies must be in place to ensure proper use Simulated electronic health record
Online learning (Jarvill et al., 2018)	Telehealth simulation Expert role modeling videos Voice thread

---

Scenario 1.3

The ANE is teaching the concept of health promotion to a group of students. One of the course objectives is "Integrate the use of technology in the care of patients, families, and communities." The ANE uses situated cognition theory and creates a simulated learning experience for the teaching strategy. This allows students to practice motivational interviewing skills and patient education with a standardized patient. The course does not have any skills laboratory or clinical hours, nor any availability for the ANE to take students to the simulation laboratory.

Consider:
1. How can the simulated learning experience happen when there is no availability in the simulation laboratory?
2. How can technology be added to the simulated learning experience to meet the course objective?
3. What other active learning strategy can replace the simulated learning experience and which learning theory would you use to support its use?

PRACTICE SKILLED ORAL AND WRITTEN (INCLUDING ELECTRONIC) COMMUNICATION THAT REFLECTS AWARENESS OF SELF AND RELATIONSHIPS WITH LEARNERS (E.G., EVALUATION, MENTORSHIP, AND SUPERVISION)

Healthy student-faculty academic relationships enhance the facilitation of learning. During the academic relationship, the ANE not only facilitates learning but evaluates, mentors, and supervises students. All entail positive, effective oral and written communication with students. Skillful communication requires ongoing practice and self-reflection to develop competency and proficiency.

The NLN calls for ANEs to practice self-awareness to recognize behaviors that impede healthy relationships with learners (NLN, 2018b). "Self-reflection and self-awareness are at the core of co-creating environments for respect and civility" (NLN, 2018b, p. 4). Self-awareness is an evolving process of self-discovery that not only includes examining one's thoughts, emotions, strengths, weaknesses, and biases but also examining the contextual factors that influence interactions with others (Rasheed, Younas, & Sundus, 2018). It is through self-awareness that ANEs commit to continuously improving relationship development and communication. Common strategies to practice self-awareness include reflection, reflective practice, and seeking feedback from others with the intent to self-improve (Rasheed et al., 2018).

COMMUNICATE EFFECTIVELY ORALLY AND IN WRITING WITH AN ABILITY TO CONVEY IDEAS IN A VARIETY OF CONTEXTS

Communication is a vital component in all areas of nursing practice, including the practice of nursing education. It is a process of transaction and message creation in a context that consists of physical space, cultural and societal values, and psychological conditions (Kourkouta & Papathanasiou, 2014). The following is a description of each context within communication, along with its considerations (Billings, 2015; Kourkouta & Papathanasiou, 2014).

Physical space	• Face-to-face: Be aware of verbal and nonverbal communication patterns (facial expressions and body position) • Distance/online: Be aware of written verbal and nonverbal communication patterns (use of capitalization, punctuation)

Cultural/societal values	• Voice pitch, tone of voice, interpersonal interaction styles, such as eye contact
	• Tips for students who are English language learners
	  • Communicate expectations both verbally and in writing.
	  • Provide key words with definitions on PowerPoint slides.
	  • Speak slowly and annunciate clearly.
	  • Avoid jargon and slang both verbally and in writing.
	  • Allow extra time for students to respond in class.

Psychological condition: calm, happy, anxious, angry, and so on	• Ensure a calming milieu.

The ANE modifies patterns of communication appropriately to effectively convey ideas. ANEs communicate many ideas with students both verbally and in writing, including—but not limited to—assignment/skill instructions, course policies, student feedback, learning objectives, and content information. Not only does clarity of all ideas facilitate learning, but clarity is a major theme in promoting nursing student engagement (Johnson-Farmer & Frenn, 2009).

MODEL REFLECTIVE THINKING PRACTICES, INCLUDING CRITICAL THINKING REFLECTIVE PRACTICE

ANEs expect students to critically reflect on their practice with the goal of self-improvement (Benner et al., 2010). However, critical reflection does not come easy to many students. Critical reflection is more than a restating of the events that happened, a common way that students reflect. It is an iterative process of learning through and from previous experiences with the intention of becoming better practitioners (Meierdirk, 2016). It is an "active, deliberate, and cognitive process" (Jacobs, 2016, p. 63). Providing the steps in the reflective process is one strategy to teach students how to become better practitioners, but this might not meet the learning needs of all students. According to constructivism, students learn through observation of others and in interaction with the "expert" (Candela, 2016). Since ANEs are the expert, it is imperative that they model critical reflective practices with their students.

Critical reflection is a constant exploration of actions, behaviors, responses, and decisions. It includes examination of situations from varying perspectives (Jacobs, 2016). Critical reflection examines outcomes resulting from actions/behaviors and asks what worked and what did not work to determine a different action/behavior that might be better to achieve the intended outcome. It is obvious that ANEs model reflective practice for students for clinical practice. However, ANEs also model critical reflection in their nursing education practice to improve as an ANE. Jacobs (2016) suggests collecting anonymous evaluations from students to gather their input on ways to better reach them. ANEs could then incorporate student feedback into the course, demonstrating flexibility and a willingness to view students' perspectives. Failure to continuously critically reflect on teaching practices results in a stagnant teaching style that most likely will impede learning for students.

Critical Thinking

Faculty must demonstrate a willingness and inclination for critical thinking and then model critical thinking for students. The literature calls this attitude "disposition toward critical thinking." Three main areas of a disposition are (a) the willingness to question everything by being a truth-seeker, inquisitive, and open-minded; (b) the desire to give structure to thinking by being analytic and systematic; and (c) being confident, yet judicious, in the face of uncertainty (Facione & Gittens, 2013). Caputi (2018) uses Tanner's (2006) four steps of clinical judgment: noticing, interpreting, responding, and reflecting. Note that reflecting, just presented, is a required skill of clinical judgment in Tanner's model. ANEs intentionally practice these skills using a clinical judgment model in addition to teaching students the model. Caputi (2018) expands on Tanner's four steps by inserting 19 critical thinking skills and strategies (also known as clinical judgment competencies). Students learn to engage in each of Tanner's steps using Caputi's clinical judgment competencies. Teaching the actual competencies is necessary for students to truly learn critical thinking in the form of clinical judgment. Following are some suggested ways:

- during faculty-to-faculty encounters (such as during councils and committee meetings)
- during faculty-to-student encounters (such as during student evaluations and clinical encounters)
- independently (such as planning teaching strategies and assessment strategies)

Social Cognitive Learning Theory states that students learn through observation of others. When ANEs model critical thinking skills with students, they experience further reinforcement of their learning (Candela, 2016).

Scenario 1.4

A student queried the ANE via the question and answer (Q&A) discussion board in the LMS in an online nursing research course. The student asked for clarification on the assignment rubric, adding the opinion that the rubric was too general and did not offer much guidance for the assignment. The ANE responded to the student's query within 24 hours to address the student's concerns. About a week later, the ANE had a phone conference with a different student about the progress of that student's assignment. During the conversation, the student communicated frustration with the same rubric for the assignment despite the ANE response on the Q&A discussion board. The ANE responded to the student by saying, "Sometimes rubrics create barriers for student creativity as they work within the confines of the rubric guidelines. Since this assignment is based on your research, I feel it is best to have a very general rubric." The student communicated understanding to the ANE's response. After the phone call, the ANE reviewed the rubric and critically reflected on the concerns of both students that occurred within a week of each other.

Consider:
1. Was there effective oral/written communication between the ANE and the students?
2. How could the communication between students and faculty have been enhanced?
3. What would you consider as you reflect on the students' concerns and the guidelines of your assignment rubric?
4. Would you consider revising the rubric to meet the students' needs now or for a future class? What other information would you want before making any revisions?
5. How would you go about gathering any further information?

CREATE OPPORTUNITIES FOR LEARNERS TO DEVELOP THEIR OWN CRITICAL THINKING SKILLS

According to Caputi (2018), nurses need to deliberately practice using critical thinking skills to improve clinical judgment and decision-making. Deliberate practice is the repetitive use of thinking skills with the intent to improve on each specific skill (Ericsson, Krampe, & Tesch-Romer, 1993). To improve, a basketball player deliberately practices the skill of free throwing. Although critical thinking is not a procedural skill, it is a cognitive skill that requires the same practice as procedural skills (Caputi, 2018). Moreover, critical thinking forms the basis for clinical reasoning and clinical judgment. If students do not have multiple opportunities to practice critical thinking, one can reason that their clinical reasoning and clinical judgment will be handicapped. Teaching assignments should require students to break down their thinking skills within the Tanner Clinical Judgment Model using Caputi's thinking skills and strategies (Caputi, 2018). Students should be required to deliberately practice each of these 19 thinking skills and strategies consistently in all settings: classroom, skills and simulation laboratories, and clinical. It is important for ANEs to know that before students can apply critical thinking (clinical judgment), they must first learn the clinical judgment model and all of its pieces, including all of the thinking skills and strategies. Once the clinical judgment model and all of the thinking skills and strategies are learned, then application with clinical judgment learning activities are planned (Caputi, 2018). The following are some strategies to promote application of critical thinking (Carvalho et al., 2017; Phillips, 2016):

- problem-based learning
- problem-based learning with concept mapping
- simulation and simulation debriefing
- intense tutoring strategies with skills laboratory session
- case studies and unfolding case studies
- questioning and Socratic questioning
- reflection and journaling
- the SEE-I method
  - Ask students to *state* it differently.
  - *Elaborate* on the topic.
  - Give an *example,* or *illustrate* it so that the meaning can be visualized.

CREATE A POSITIVE LEARNING ENVIRONMENT THAT FOSTERS A FREE EXCHANGE OF IDEAS

Academic incivility is any speech or behavior by students or faculty that negatively impacts students or faculty, weakens relationships, and compromises the teaching-learning process (Palumbo, 2018). ANEs ensure that learning environments are free of negative behaviors so that students feel safe to share ideas without fear of ridicule/judgment from their peers or the ANE. Table 1.5 presents a list of uncivil behaviors exhibited by ANEs and students that compromise a safe learning environment (Clark, 2017; Luparell & Conner, 2016).

The following are some strategies that ANEs can use to prevent uncivil behaviors, thereby fostering positive learning environments (Clark, 2017; Lerret & Frenn, 2011; Luparell & Conner, 2016; Palumbo, 2018).

Table 1.5

Uncivil Behaviors of ANEs and Students

ANE Uncivil Behaviors	Student Uncivil Behaviors
Unresponsive to student needs/not being available outside of class/showing disinterest in students	Talking badly about instructors
Unprepared to teach	Cell phone use in class
Challenging other instructor's knowledge	Challenging the instructor
Attempting to "weed out" certain students	Cheating/plagiarism
Setting students up to fail	Tardiness/leaving class early/sleeping in class
Defensive behavior	Not listening/talking in class
Rude/condescending remarks/name calling/scare tactics	Sarcastic remarks
Violations of due process	Uncooperative
Unexpected course changes	Alcohol/drug possession
Loss of patience	Physical/verbal abuse
Presenting lectures too fast with little to no student involvement	Eating/drinking in class
	Intimidation/stalking

- Explicitly describe appropriate behaviors to students on the first day of class and clearly identify goals and expectations in the syllabus.
- Be assertive and inform students of the student conduct policies of the institution.
- Provide open communication about course assignments, decision-making, and grading.
- Establish a trusting environment.
- Inform students on the purpose of constructive feedback and provide effective feedback for student behaviors.
- Provide an educational module on incivility and ways to positively intervene.
- Remind students of appropriate behavior within an educational framework.
- Ask the disruptive student to leave class and file an official complaint about the student's behavior.
- Consult with an experienced faculty member for ways to manage uncivil student and faculty behavior.
- Maintain self-awareness of feelings when engaging with students.
- When discussing uncivil behaviors with students, be cognizant of different perspectives related to what constitutes uncivil behaviors that may differ between the ANE and the students.
- Listen and communicate value and respect to students, and provide feedback in a way that encourages rather than demeans students.
- Maintain a strong social presence in the online learning environment:
  - instructor-made short videos/podcasts
  - timely responses to student discussion forum posts and emails
  - individualized feedback and encouragement

SHOW ENTHUSIASM FOR TEACHING, LEARNING, AND THE NURSING PROFESSION THAT INSPIRES AND MOTIVATES STUDENTS

Enthusiasm is a key characteristic of becoming an effective teacher. If teachers do not exhibit excitement for the profession or for teaching and learning, then how can they motivate students to persevere through the learning process while mastering challenging knowledge, skills, and attitudes needed to become safe nurses at all levels? Faculty are better able to engage students in learning when faculty show enjoyment and interest for the subject matter being taught; this, in turn, motivates and inspires students (Lerret & Frenn, 2011; Sedden & Clark, 2016). How do teachers display enthusiasm and passion? ANEs demonstrate enthusiasm by exhibiting energy and excitement for the subject matter and varying tonal inflection with consistency between facial expressions and verbal messages. When students perceive that faculty are passionate about the learning potential of each student, students are inspired to achieve more (Lerret & Frenn, 2011).

DEMONSTRATE PERSONAL ATTRIBUTES THAT FACILITATE LEARNING (E.G., CARING, CONFIDENCE, PATIENCE, INTEGRITY, RESPECT, AND FLEXIBILITY)

Caring is a core value of nursing and includes behaviors of sharing self, developing trust, instilling confidence, demonstrating flexibility, and creating a respectful and supportive learning environment (Fifer, 2019). Student-faculty trust, along with its related characteristics, impacts student success in higher education (Varagona & Hold, 2019). Not only do caring behaviors positively influence the student-faculty relationship and student success, students can learn these behaviors through caring interactions with faculty (Fifer, 2019). Students perceive faculty to be trustworthy when they give of themselves, are competent, and have integrity. ANEs should consistently role model these behaviors in all learning environments. Some strategies that ANEs can implement to role model caring behaviors, including trustworthiness, are as follows (Fifer, 2019; Gaudine & Moralejo, 2011; Varagona & Hold, 2019):

- Foster engagement in the learning environment and ask for ongoing feedback from students.
- Have students complete a learning styles inventory to consider the needs of each student.
- Be competent and passionate about the subject material.
- Write good test items.
- Be receptive and available to meet with students individually or in groups; schedule virtual office hours in the evening using the phone or video conferencing.
- Be compassionate, open-minded, and open to influence.
- Actively listen to students.
- Be accountable and acknowledge errors.
- Show respect and avoid being judgmental.
- Maintain congruence with verbal and nonverbal communication.
- Help students be successful, boost student self-confidence, and demonstrate a personal interest in their success.
- Share power by including students in developing some course policies/due dates/acceptable topics for projects/rubrics/discussion guidelines/learning outcomes.
- Use audio or video streamed lectures on the LMS for access to content for convenience.
- Be truthful, fair, and honorable in principles, intentions, and actions.

ANEs consistently demonstrate these behaviors to maintain the trust of students. When trust is lost, it is difficult to regain (Varagona & Hold, 2019).

Scenario 1.5

An online student posted the following question to a discussion board regarding an assignment: "I'm a little confused about how to do the voice thread 5-minute pitch. Is the Power-Point poster going to show up 'in total' on the full screen? Or will we have to zoom into one section, like Prezi? Also, the information I've read says the font size needs to be >75, which I understand for real posters, but I'm not sure how it translates for our project. Is there an example from a previous class to get some clarification?" The response posted by the ANE was: "I wish I could provide a previous example but unfortunately there is no way to hide the student's identity so I would need their permission to share it. However, I can create an example using one of my posters that I have presented. I will let everyone know when that is ready to view. This presentation will be just like your journal presentation assignment."

Consider:
1. How is this faculty member demonstrating enthusiasm for teaching?
2. Do you recognize any caring attributes in the faculty response? Is this brief response motivating for students?
3. How does this response create a positive learning environment?
4. How would you handle the student's query regarding the assignment to meet your goal of demonstrating enthusiasm, caring, and a positive learning environment?

Furthermore, students develop preconceived thoughts about faculty from peers. To prevent students from forming preconceived thoughts, avoid behaviors that are not consistent with the strategies just discussed so that students hear only positive comments from their peers.

RESPOND EFFECTIVELY TO UNEXPECTED EVENTS THAT AFFECT INSTRUCTION

Unexpected events are bound to happen during the academic year. Some examples of unexpected events include student physical or mental illness, illness or death in a student's family, school closings related to weather emergencies, or school violence. These unexpected events can impede learning for individual students in the case of personal unexpected events or for groups of students in the case of weather emergencies. Missed classes, exams, skills practice, or even clinical experiences can cause anxiety for students. This is the perfect opportunity for ANEs to use caring behaviors. Effective responses to such events assist in maintaining students' positive emotions, which can build or reinforce trust in faculty (Varagona & Hold, 2019). In these circumstances, the ANE works with students and is reasonably flexible in making adjustments to assignment due dates, exam dates, clinical makeup dates, and so on. These behaviors reinforce to students that faculty care about their success (Fifer, 2019). Schools of nursing have adopted emergency plans to put into place if a weather-related event causes an unexpected, unplanned closure of the school. School violence also requires faculty to change educational plans in a quick fashion. No matter what the event, faculty must always be prepared and able to respond effectively to unexpected events that affect instruction.

Develop Collegial Working Relationships with Clinical Agency Personnel to Promote Positive Learning

There are primarily two important reasons for the development of collegial working relationships with clinical agencies. First, the shortage of clinical sites is evident in nursing education (Kovner & Djukic, 2009). Once a clinical site has been procured, ANEs deliberately foster effective working relationships to retain clinical practice sites, enhancing the educational experience for students (Gubrud, 2016). Second, uncivil behaviors toward nursing students by clinical agency staff can occur. This not only leads to feelings of stress, but students can learn these negative behaviors from agency staff (Yang-Heui & Choi, 2019). Creating a positive working relationship with agency staff may assist in preventing incivility toward students. ANEs help clinical agencies realize the mutually beneficial effects of the clinical agency-nursing program partnership. Some recommendations for developing collegial working relationships include the following:

- Ongoing effective communication with agency staff related to:
  - goals, competencies, outcomes
  - level of students
  - practice expectations
  - clinical schedule
- Understanding the agency environment and the agency staff roles
- Modifying teaching approaches to the individual agency situations
- Ensuring orientation for students
- Encouraging students to engage with agency staff early in the clinical experience

ANEs gather feedback on the experiences from students, clinical administrators, and staff for the purpose of implementing changes that will improve the experience for all (Lloyd-Penza, Rose, & Roach, 2019). This strengthens partnerships, supports student learning needs, and improves student experiences.

Use Knowledge of Evidence-Based Practice to Instruct Learners

As discussed earlier in this chapter, ANEs use research to inform their teaching and learning process (NLN, 2016a). Evidence-based practice is a lifelong problem-solving approach to delivering quality health care integrating well-designed studies, patient preferences and values, and the clinician's expertise (Melnyk, Gallagher-Ford, Long, & Fineout-Overholt, 2014). This definition is clinically focused on patient care. The ultimate goal of nursing education is quality patient care (NLN, 2016a). Therefore, ANEs use their knowledge of evidence-based practice to inform nursing education to prepare students with the knowledge, skills, and attitudes needed to deliver quality patient care. ANEs shift their thinking from implementing strategies based on "this is how we have done it" to searching the literature for well-designed studies in teaching strategies, integrating student preferences and values, and the educator's expertise. Melnyk et al. (2014) identified 24 evidence-based competencies for advanced practice nurses. The following competencies have been modified to align with the advanced practice role of the nurse educator:

- Questions educational practice to improve quality instruction that ultimately improves quality care
- Describes the educational problem
- Formulates the educational question in the PICOT format (population, intervention, comparison intervention or group, outcome, time)
- Systematically conducts an exhaustive search for external evidence to answer the educational question
- Critically appraises relevant preappraised evidence (e.g., educational standards) and primary studies, including evaluation and synthesis

- Integrates a body of external and internal evidence to plan evidence-based decisions about educational interventions
- Leads faculty teams in applying synthesized evidence to initiate educational decisions and practice changes to improve instruction with the ultimate goal of quality nursing care
- Implements the practice change based on evidence, educational expertise, and student preferences to improve student learning
- Generates internal evidence through outcomes management and implementation projects with the purpose of integrating best practice
- Formulates evidence-based policies for the nursing program
- Participates in generation of external evidence
- Mentors others in evidence-based decision-making and the evidence-based process
- Implements strategies to sustain a culture of evidence-based practice
- Communicates best evidence to individuals and colleagues

Demonstrates Ability to Teach Clinical Skills

ANEs teach clinical skills in places that allow students to interact with patients and families for the purpose of acquiring the cognitive, psychomotor, and affective skills needed for professional nursing practice (Gubrud, 2016). Therefore, clinical skills can be taught in the following environments:

- clinical learning resource centers (skills laboratories)
- simulation laboratories
- virtual clinical environments
- acute and transitional care environments
- community-based environments

Effective clinical teaching requires using multiple instructional techniques and strategies, allowing for successful learning of clinical skills. To effectively teach clinical skills, ANEs need to (Girija, 2012; Gubrud, 2016; Valiee, Glorokh, Khaledi, & Garibi, 2016):

- Demonstrate professional competence.
  - Be confident with knowledge/skills/attitudes.
    - Convey knowledge in an understandable way to facilitate transfer of theory to practice.
      - Ask students questions that require analysis/synthesis.
      - Have students provide peer or patient teaching.
      - Assist students in recognizing salient clues in clinical.
    - Be competent in clinical skills.
    - Know the learners individually.
  - Be accessible to students in clinical.
  - Evaluate student performance.
    - Be objective and fair.
    - Provide timely constructive and specific feedback.
  - Use effective communication and interpersonal skills.
    - Clearly inform students of goals and expectations.
    - Interact with students during the clinical day.
    - Collaborate with other disciplines for learning experiences.
    - Be open-minded and nonjudgmental.
    - Correct mistakes without belittling.

- Build relationships with students.
  - Encourage students to ask questions.
  - Permit expression of feelings.
  - Use a mentoring approach with students.
  - Support students to promote their independence and self-confidence.
- Demonstrate personal attributes.
  - Be approachable, honest, and direct.
  - Demonstrate patience.
  - Show enthusiasm.
  - Be well prepared, organized, and self-confident.

Act as a Role Model in Practice Settings

As discussed throughout this chapter, ANEs facilitate learning of the required professional knowledge, skills, and attitudes for students to provide safe, quality nursing care. Facilitation of learning does not occur only with the various evidence-based teaching strategies presented in this chapter but also when nursing students interact with and observe behaviors of their ANE. Grounded in Social Cognitive Theory, ANEs facilitate learning by students observing them as models of professional behavior (Candela, 2016). Nursing students have a number of role models throughout an academic program. They experience a variety of faculty and work with a variety of staff nurses, preceptors, and interprofessional practitioners in the clinical practice environment. Because students are exposed to a variety of role models, they will likely observe positive and negative behaviors (Reader, Hamshire, & Chambers, 2017). When students are exposed to negative behaviors, they are at a high risk for emulating those behaviors, leading to poor outcomes for themselves and others. This makes it extremely important for ANEs to consistently model positive professional behaviors.

ANEs need to be consciously aware that their professional behaviors in the clinical, classroom, and skills and simulation laboratory settings are always being observed by nursing students. Nursing students perceive ANEs to be positive role models when they demonstrate clinical competence, are effective teachers, and relate to students on an interpersonal level (Reader et al., 2017). Positive professional role modeling behavior is an effective way to facilitate learning for nursing students.

Scenario 1.6

A nursing student who is planning to administer medications to a patient tells the clinical instructor that the patient's chart documents an allergy to beta blockers. The student says "The patient is prescribed metoprolol, which is a beta blocker." The ANE says, "That is a great assessment and you really know your medications! What is your plan?" The student states "I need to speak with this patient's nurse." After consulting with the patient's nurse, the student informs the instructor that the patient has been given the beta blocker for quite some time and the information in the patient's chart is wrong. The student tells the instructor, "The nurse said I can go ahead and give the medication."

Consider:
1. What will you do to be a role model for this student?
2. How can this concern be addressed with the clinical agency while maintaining a collegial working relationship?
3. What actions would you take to build a healthy relationship with the student and foster enthusiasm for learning?

Table 1.6

Uncivil Behaviors of ANEs and Students in the Online Learning Environment

ANE Online Uncivil Behaviors	Student Online Uncivil Behaviors
Acting disinterested	Challenging authority or testing the instructor's knowledge
Making snide remarks or invalidating student remarks	
	Making hostile and offensive remarks
Humiliating students	Missing deadlines
Having unrealistic expectations	Dominating discussions or reluctant to participate
Sending inappropriate emails	Sending inappropriate emails
Exerting power	Belittling others
Threatening to fail students	Demanding special treatment

FOSTER A SAFE LEARNING ENVIRONMENT

The final role of the ANE is to effectively facilitate learning that aligns directly with creating positive learning environments so that students are free to exchange ideas, a role discussed earlier in this chapter. When the learning environment is ridden with uncivil behaviors, the teaching-learning process will be affected (Palumbo, 2018). There are multiple environments in which ANEs facilitate learning: the classroom, skills and simulation laboratories, and clinical. ANEs foster safe learning environments in each of these settings. Previously in this chapter, it was discussed how ANEs or students may exhibit uncivil behaviors (see Table 1.5). The same strategies recommended to create a positive environment also foster a safe environment.

Online learning is an environment where incivility is also possible by both the ANE and students (Donathan, Hands, & Dotson, 2017). Table 1.6 presents uncivil ANE and student behaviors in the online learning environment (Donathan et al., 2017).

As discussed earlier in this chapter, the ANE communicates effectively in writing using respectful, civil language (Donathan et al., 2017). Written communication is especially important when facilitating learning in the online environment. This is an excellent opportunity for the ANE to practice reflective thinking when students are not participating according to expectations. Collecting frequent anonymous surveys through the LMS helps the ANE gather data for self-reflection and improvement (Donathan et al., 2017).

Strategies to prevent uncivil student behaviors in the online learning environment include the following (Donathan et al., 2017):

• Clearly describe student expectations in the course syllabus.
• Distribute a handout on respectful "netiquette" behaviors and consequences of not following these behaviors.
• Introduce self and share credentials and experience.
• Provide an "ice breaker" activity in the first week discussion board for students.
• Provide frequent feedback.
• Inform students when and how they will receive feedback.
• Keep students engaged in the course with active learning strategies.
• Encourage respectful debate of topics while reinforcing that attacking students is inappropriate behavior.

SUMMARY

This chapter presented current research on ways the ANE facilitates learning. Students absorb information best when they participate in a variety of learning experiences and use their natural disposition for learning. A variety of contexts support learning, although no one is superior over another. ANEs are encouraged to shift from a teacher-centered environment, conveying an ever-growing body of content, to a student-centered environment, teaching concepts with application and helping students learn how to find information independently and give it meaning. Actively engaging students in the learning experience rather than having them passively listen to a lecture provides the framework for collaboration, teamwork, communication, and critical thinking. By eliminating bias from the educational environment, faculty establish a milieu where ethnically and racially diverse students, genders, and differing age groups can thrive.

ANEs have dual responsibility. They monitor both the clinical and educational literature to remain current in their nursing clinical practice and their nursing education practice. They search databases that feature pedagogical research to ground their teaching and use innovative strategies to facilitate learning using the best available evidence. Finally, ANEs are effective role models and should never underestimate the influence of their professional behaviors on student learning.

Practice Test Questions

1. The nursing instructor is planning a learning strategy to engage students in critical thinking. Which teaching strategy best fosters the student's ability to engage in critical thinking?
   A. Lecture with PowerPoint slides about the nursing interventions required for postpartum hemorrhage
   B. Student observation of the mother-baby nurse providing care to postpartum patients in the clinical setting
   C. Small group concept map of a case study of a patient who is in labor and having late decelerations
   D. Students playing a *Jeopardy* game, with each category related to a common concept of the childbearing family

2. A novice faculty member is planning evidence-based active learning strategies that require higher-order thinking. Which statement by a novice faculty member requires further guidance from the mentoring faculty member?
   A. "My students will be working on a case study during class today."
   B. "I found this great YouTube video that shows how the heart pumps blood."
   C. "The discussion board works great for students to journal postclinical."
   D. "I am going to have students practice sterile glove technique in the skills laboratory."

3. A nurse educator is teaching graduate level students in an asynchronous online course and wants to integrate teaching strategies that align with Adult Learning Theory. Which teaching strategy will the nurse educator choose?
   A. Podcast lecture
   B. Discussion board case study
   C. Role play
   D. Personal response system activity

4. Which statement by the academic nurse educator best demonstrates effective communication with a student who is an English language learner?
   A. "Please be sure to review how the heart pumps blood."
   B. "What is your patient's crit value?"
   C. "Tell me the six rights to medication administration."
   D. "How will the patient smoking weed impact your care?"

5. What is the best way to communicate assignment instructions when working with students with diverse learning styles in the online learning environment?
   A. Send individual emails to students.
   B. Post the written instructions to the discussion board.
   C. Provide an example assignment along with the instructions.
   D. Upload a voiceover PowerPoint of the instructions.

6. The nurse faculty member is preparing to deliver a poor student evaluation. Which strategy will best prepare the faculty member to promote a healthy academic relationship before meeting with the student?
   A. Use guided imagery considering thoughts and feelings of self and student.
   B. Role play the conversation with a fellow colleague.
   C. Write a list of the strengths and weaknesses of the student performance.
   D. Ensure that the physical meeting space is completely private.

7. The program chair is reviewing student course evaluations. Which written student comment best demonstrates faculty expertise in facilitating learning?
   A. "There was always extensive information on the PowerPoint slides! I didn't need to take notes and I was able to really concentrate on what was being taught."
   B. "The teacher was kind and gentle and was always so prepared for class. I was excited about the technology used in class."
   C. "He gave prompt feedback to written assignments and quickly answered my emails. I found him to be quite engaged with the class!"
   D. "Somehow she managed to make concept mapping a fun learning experience despite the difficulty level. It made me want to dive right in!"

8. Which strategy best engages millennial students and helps them practice decision-making?
   A. Include YouTube videos and photos on PowerPoint slides.
   B. Use a personal response system with NCLEX-style questions.
   C. Use Socratic questioning with the students.
   D. Ask students to write practice NCLEX-style questions on covered content.

9. A nursing student is worried about missing the next scheduled exam to attend a family member's funeral. Which method is the most effective way for the nurse educator to respond to this event?
   A. Mutually agree on a date/time within one week of the funeral for the student to take the exam.
   B. Offer the student the opportunity to take the exam the day before the funeral.
   C. Ask the student how close a relationship the student had with the family member.
   D. Bring a condolence card to class and ask the other students in the class to sign the card.

10. Which evidence-based active learning strategy best assists students to function as a team, appreciate team differences, and use critical thinking skills?
    A. Socratic questioning
    B. Collaborative testing
    C. Case studies
    D. Creating algorithms

11. A faculty member notices that students are unprepared for class and use their cell phones or computers for activities unrelated to the lecture topic. Which is the best strategy to remedy the situation at this time?
    A. Stop the lecture and politely ask students to pay attention, then start again.
    B. Continue the lecture and ignore the behaviors, since they are not disturbing other students.

C. Involve the students by asking them to use their cell phones to look up information.

D. Review organizational values with the students and remind them of their professional responsibility.

12. Which statement by the novice nurse educator demonstrates the need for further mentoring regarding the use of evidence-based practice for teaching nursing students?

A. "I think I am going to implement teaching strategies that have quite a bit of literature that supports a positive learning environment."

B. "The students complained about the amount of work when I started flipping the class but their test scores significantly improved!"

C. "Teaching nursing research online can be quite challenging. I found a few articles discussing the value of student virtual poster presentations."

D. "Students consistently ask for more lecture time in class. Since they really don't like the group work, I plan to increase the amount of lecture I provide."

13. The nurse educator's philosophy of education aligns with Social Cognitive Theory. Which teaching strategy best aligns with this theory?

A. Role model appropriate technique and behavior in clinical.

B. Have students individually practice physical assessment in the skills laboratory.

C. Use personal response systems to survey the class in lecture.

D. Create a podcast lecture for the LMS.

14. Which statement by the nurse educator best demonstrates the ability to meet the diverse learning needs of students?

A. "The research shows that millennial learners like technology so I think we should adopt the policy of only using e-books."

B. "I like to assess which students have health care work experience before assigning students to groups for a case study assignment."

C. "It is beneficial to have students view an expert perform a skill and then have them practice using the skills checklist."

D. "Students really enjoy playing *Jeopardy* in my class. It keeps them really engaged!"

15. The nursing student asks the clinical instructor why the patient's diuretic is being held for a high potassium level. How will the nurse educator best respond?

A. Tell the student to ask the patient's nurse.

B. Teach the student about potassium-wasting diuretics.

C. Have the student investigate and report in post-conference.

D. Review all of the patient's medications with the student to find the answer.

16. Which action by the nurse educator best promotes an effective clinical experience for both the clinical site and the students?

A. Telling the clinical site the date/time for clinical site orientation

B. Communicating the clinical objectives with the unit manager

C. Having students administer medication with their assigned staff nurse

D. Asking the charge nurse to make patient assignments for students

17. The nurse educator assesses that ¼ of the students in the lecture class are from the baby boomer generation. Which teaching strategy is most acceptable to students in the baby boomer generation?
A. Incorporate some lecture with PowerPoint.
B. Include the use of drug guides accessed with mobile devices.
C. Add virtual simulation for homework assignments.
D. Use more concept maps during class time.

18. The nursing instructor expects students in a pathophysiology course to be able to correlate the physiological changes experienced by complex medical patients with their clinical manifestations and complications. Which strategy should the instructor choose to best foster this type of critical thinking?
A. Use Socratic questioning to help students determine what to assess.
B. Lecture about disease manifestations and physiological changes.
C. Assign students to write a one-minute paper on disease complications.
D. Show a 20-minute movie about a pertinent clinical case.

19. An experienced faculty member is mentoring a novice faculty member with facilitating a simulated learning experience. Which action by the novice faculty member requires further guidance by the experienced faculty member?
A. Provide the objectives of the simulated learning experience to the students in prebriefing.
B. Review expectations of appropriate student conduct during the simulated learning experience.
C. Request student volunteers for the roles of the nurse and family member.
D. Highlight students' errors during debriefing so that they can learn from their mistakes.

20. The nurse educator is planning activities for the first day of clinical in critical care with a new group of students. Which activity best motivates students to learn and encourage learning through role modeling?
A. Ensure that the clinical agency staff provide an orientation to the unit for students.
B. Identify the list of skills that students will be able to perform at the clinical site.
C. Share personal credentials and passion for caring for patients in critical care.
D. Provide written documentation of clinical objectives and expectations during clinical.

References

Alexander, G. R. (2016). Multicultural education in nursing. In D. M. Billings & J. A. Halstead (Eds.), *Teaching in nursing: A guide for faculty* (5th ed., pp. 263–281). St. Louis, MO: Elsevier.

Aljezawi, M., & Albashtawy, M. (2015). Quiz game teaching format versus didactic lectures. *British Journal of Nursing, 24*(2), 86–92.

Badowski, D., Horsley, T. L., Rossler, K. L., Mariani, B., & Gonzalez, L. (2018). Electronic charting during simulation: A descriptive study. *CIN: Computers, Informatics, Nursing, 36*(9), 430–437. doi: 10.1097/CIN0000000000000457

Benner, P., Sutphen, M., Leonard, V., & Day, L. (2010). *Educating nurses: A call for radical transformation.* San Francisco, CA: Jossey-Bass.

Betihavas, V., Bridgman, H., Kornhaber, R., & Cross, M. (2016). The evidence for 'flipping out': A systematic review of the flipped classroom in nursing education. *Nurse Education Today, 38*, 15–21. http://dx.doi.org/10.1016/j.nedt.2015.12.010

Billings, D. M. (2015). Culturally and linguistically responsive teaching: Part I. *The Journal of Continuing Education in Nursing, 46*(2), 62–64. doi:10.3928/00220124-20150121-14

Braungart, M. M., Braungart, R. G., & Gramet, P. R. (2019). Applying learning theories to healthcare practice. In S. B. Bastable (Ed.), *Nurse as educator* (5th ed., pp. 69–115). Burlington, MA: Jones & Barlett Learning.

Breytenbach, C., Ham-Baloyi, W., & Jordan, P. (2017). An integrative literature review of evidence-based teaching strategies for nurse educators. *Nursing Education Perspectives, 38*(4), 193–197. doi: 10.1097/01.NEP.0000000000000181

Candela, L. (2016). Theoretical foundations of teaching and learning. In D. M. Billings & J. A. Halstead (Eds.), *Teaching in nursing: A guide for faculty* (5th ed., pp. 211–229). St. Louis, MO: Elsevier.

Caputi, L. (2018). *Think like a nurse handbook*. Rolling Meadows, IL: Windy City Publishers.

Caputi, L., & Frank, B. (2019). Competency I: Facilitate learning. In J. A. Halstead (Ed.), *NLN core competencies for nurse educators: A decade of influence* (pp. 17–43). Washington, DC: National League for Nursing.

Carvalho, D., Azevedo, I. C., Cruz, G. K. P., Mafra, G. A. C., Rego, A. L. C., Vitor, A.F., ... Ferreira Junior, M. A. (2017). Strategies used for the promotion of critical thinking in nursing undergraduate education: A systematic review. *Nurse Education Today, 57*, 103–107. http://dx.doi.org/10.1016/j.nedt.2017.07.010

Clark, K. R. (2017). Managing the higher education classroom. *Radiologic Technology, 89*(2), 210–213.

Donathan, L. N., Hands, M., & Dotson, A. T. (2017). Minimizing incivility in the online classroom. *Radiologic Technology, 89*(1), 88–91.

Efstathiou, N., & Bailey, C. (2012). Promoting active learning using Audience Response System in large bioscience classes. *Nurse Education Today, 32*(1), 91–95. doi: 10.1016/j.nedt.2011.01.017

Ericsson, K. A., Krampe, T. T., & Tesch-Romer, C. (1993). The role of deliberate practice in the acquisition of expert performance. *Psychological Review, 100*(3), 363–406. doi: 10.1037/0033-295X.100.3.363

Facione, P., & Gittens, C. (2013). *Think critically*. Upper Saddle River, NJ: Prentice Hall.

Fifer, P. (2019). Associate degree nursing students' perceptions of instructor caring. *Teaching and Learning in Nursing, 14*, 103–110. https://doi.org/10.1016/jteln.2018.12.006

Gaudine, A. P., & Moralejo, D. G. (2011). What can faculty members and programs do to improve students' learning? *ISRN Nursing, 2011*. doi:10.5402/2011/649431

Girija, K. M. (2012). Effective clinical instructor: A step toward excellence in clinical teaching. *International Journal of Nursing Education, 4*(1), 25–27.

Gruendemann, B. J. (2011). Nursing student experiences with face-to-face learning. *Journal of Nursing Education, 50*(12), 676–680. doi:10.3928/01484834-20110930-02

Gubrud, P. (2016). Teaching in the clinical setting. In D. M. Billings & J. A. Halstead (Eds.), *Teaching in nursing: A guide for faculty* (5th ed., pp. 282–303). St. Louis, MO: Elsevier.

Hayden, J. K., Smiley, R. A., Alexander, M., Kardong-Edgren, S., & Jeffries, P. R. (2014). Supplement: The NCSBN National Simulation Study: A longitudinal, randomized, controlled study replacing clinical hours with simulation in prelicensure nursing education. *Journal of Nursing Regulation, 5*(2), S1–S64. doi:10.1016/S2155-8256(15)30062-4

INACSL Standards Committee (2016). INACSL standards of best practice: Simulation^SM Simulation glossary. *Clinical Simulation in Nursing, 12*(S), S39–S47. http://dx.doi.org/10.1016/j.ecns.2016.09.012

Institute of Medicine (2011). *The future of nursing: Leading change, advancing health*. Washington, DC: National Academies Press.

Jacobs, S. (2016). Reflective learning, reflective practice. *Nursing 2016, 46*(5), 62–64. doi: 10.1097/01.NURSE.0000482278.79660.f2

Jarvill, M., Kelly, S., & Krebs, H. (2018). Effect of expert role modeling on skill performance in simulation. *Clinical Simulation in Nursing, 24*(C), 25–29. https://doi.org/10.1016/j.ecns.2018.08.005

Johnson-Farmer, B. J., & Frenn, M. (2009). Teaching excellence: What great teachers teach us. *Journal of Professional Nursing, 25*(5), 267–272. doi: 10.1016/j.profnurs.2009.01.020

Kalb, K. A., O'Conner-Von, S. K., Brockway, C., Rierson, C. L., & Sendelbach, S. (2015). Evidence-based teaching practice in nursing education: Faculty perspectives and practices. *Nursing Education Perspectives, 36*(4), 212–219. doi: 10.5480/14-1472

Kitchie, S. (2019). Determinants of learning. In S. B. Bastable (Ed.), *Nurse as educator* (5th ed., pp. 119–168). Burlington, MA: Jones & Barlett Learning.

Knowles, M. S. (1980). *The modern practice of adult education*. Chicago, IL: Follett.

Kourkouta, L., & Papathanasiou, I. V. (2014). Communication in nursing practice. *Materia Socio-Medica, 26*(1), 65–67. doi:10.5455/msm.2014.26.65-67

Kovner, C., & Djukic, M. (2009). The nursing career process from application through the first 2 years of employment. *Journal of Professional Nursing, 25*(4), 197–203. doi:10.1016/j.profnurs.2009.05.002

Lerret, S. M., & Frenn, M. (2011). Challenge with care: Reflections on teaching excellence. *Journal of Professional Nursing, 27*(6), 378–384. doi:10.1016/j.profnurs.2011.04.014

Lloyd-Penza, M., Rose, A., & Roach, A. (2019). Using feedback to improve clinical education of nursing students in an academic-practice partnership. *Teaching and Learning in Nursing 14*, 125–127. https://doi.org/10.1016/j.teln2018.12.007

Luparell, S., & Conner, J. R., (2016). Managing student incivility and misconduct in the learning environment. In D. M. Billings & J. A. Halstead (Eds.), *Teaching in nursing: A guide for faculty* (5th ed., pp. 15–34). St. Louis, MO: Elsevier.

Mareno, N., Bremner, M., & Emerson, C. (2010). The use of Audience Response Systems in nursing education: Best practice guidelines. *International Journal of Nursing Education Scholarship, 7*(1), Article 32. Retrieved from http://dx.doi.org/10.2202/1548-923X.2049

McAfooes, J. (2016). Teaching and learning in online learning communities. In D. M. Billings & J. A. Halstead (Eds.), *Teaching in nursing: A guide for faculty* (5th ed., pp. 357–384). St. Louis, MO: Elsevier.

Meierdirk, S. (2016). Is reflective practice an essential component of becoming a professional teacher? *Reflective Practice, 17*(3), 369–378. http://dx.doi.org/10.1080/14623943.2016.1169169.

Melnyk, B. M., Gallagher-Ford, L., Long, L. E., & Fineout-Overholt, E. (2014). The establishment of evidence-based practice competencies for practicing registered nurses and advanced practice nurses in real-world clinical setting: Proficiencies to improve healthcare quality, reliability, patient outcomes, and costs. *Worldviews on Evidence-Based Nursing, 11*(1), 5–15. https://doi.org/10.1111/wvn.12021 |

Mueller, C. (2016). Service learning: Developing values, cultural competence, social responsibility, and global awareness. In D. M. Billings & J. A. Halstead (Eds.), *Teaching in nursing: A guide for faculty* (5th ed., pp. 197–210). St. Louis, MO: Elsevier.

National League for Nursing (2006). *Excellence in nursing education model.* New York: Author.

National League for Nursing (2015). A vision for the changing faculty role: Preparing students for the technological world of health care. *NLN Vision Series.* Retrieved from http://www.nln.org/docs/default-source/about/nln-vision-series-(position-statements)/a-vision-for-the-changing-faculty-role-preparing-students-for-the-technological-world-of-health-care.pdf?sfvrsn=0.

National League for Nursing (2016a). A vision for advancing the science of nursing education: The NLN nursing education research priorities (2016–2019). *NLN Vision Series.* Retrieved from http://www.nln.org/docs/default-source/about/nln-vision-series-(position-statements)/a-vision-for-advancing-the-science.pdf?sfvrsn=2.

National League for Nursing (2016b). Percentage of minorities enrolled in basic RN programs by race-ethnicity: 2014 and 2016. *NLN DataView^{TM}.* Retrieved from http://www.nln.org/docs/default-source/newsroom/nursing-education-statistics/percentage-of-minorities-enrolled-in-basic-rn-programs-by-race-ethnicity-2014-and-2016-(pdf).pdf?sfvrsn=0.

National League for Nursing (2016c). Percentage of students enrolled in nursing programs by sex and program type, 2016. *NLN DataView^{TM}.* Retrieved from http://www.nln.org/docs/default-source/newsroom/nursing-education-statistics/percentage-of-students-enrolled-in-nursing-program-by-sex-and-program-type-2016-(pdf).pdf?sfvrsn=0.

National League for Nursing (2016d). Percentage of students enrolled by age and program type, 2015–2016. *NLN DataView^{TM}.* Retrieved from http://www.nln.org/docs/default-source/newsroom/nursing-education-statistics/percentage-of-students-enrolled-by-age-and-program-type-2016-(pdf).pdf?sfvrsn=0.

National League for Nursing (2018a). *Certified Nurse Educator® 2018 Candidate Handbook.* Retrieved from http://www.nln.org/docs/default-source/default-document-library/cne-handbookb203c85c78366c709642ff00005f0421.pdf?sfvrsn.

National League for Nursing (2018b). Creating community to build a civil and healthy academic work environment. *NLN Vision Series.* Retrieved from http://www.nln.org/docs/default-source/professional-development-programs/vision-statement-a-vision-for-creating-community-to-build-a-civil-and-healthy.pdf?sfvrsn=8http://www.nln.org/docs/default-source/professional-development-programs/vision-statement-a-vision-for-creating-community-to-build-a-civil-and-healthy.pdf?sfvrsn=10&pdf=VisionSeries-CreatingCommunity.

Njie-Carr, V. P. K., Ludeman, E., Lee, M. C., Dordunoo, D., Trocky, N. M., & Jenkins, L. S. (2017). An integrative review of flipped classroom teaching models in nursing education. *Journal of Professional Nursing, 33*(2), 133–144. http://dx.doi.org/10.1016/j.profnurs.2016.07.001

Oermann, M. H., & Gaberson, K. B. (2017). *Evaluation and testing in nursing education* (5th ed.). New York, NY: Springer Publishing.

Palumbo, R. (2018). Incivility in nursing education: An intervention. *Nurse Education Today, 66,* 143–148. https://doi.org/10.1016/j.nedt.2018.03.024

Paul, R., & Elder, L. (2013). The standards for thinking. In R. Paul & L. Elder, *Critical thinking: Tools for taking charge of your professional and personal life* (2nd ed., pp. 98–129). Upper Saddle River, NJ: Pearson Prentice Hall.

Phillips, J. M. (2016). Strategies to promote student engagement and active learning. In D. M. Billings & J. A. Halstead (Eds.), *Teaching in nursing: A guide for faculty* (5th ed., pp. 245–262). St. Louis, MO: Elsevier.

Popkess, A. M., & Frey, J. L. (2016). Strategies to support diverse learning needs of students. In D. M. Billings & J. A. Halstead (Eds.), *Teaching in nursing: A guide for faculty* (5th ed., pp. 15–34). St. Louis, MO: Elsevier, Inc.

Ramsden, P. (2013). Learning from student's perspective. In *Learning to teach in higher education* (3rd ed., pp. 62–83). London: Routledge.

Rasheed, S. P., Younas, A., & Sundus, A. (2018). Self-awareness in nursing: A scoping review. *Journal of Clinical Nursing, 28,* 762–774. doi: 10.1111/jocn.14708

Reader, K. J., Hamshire, C., & Chambers, A. (2017). The influence of role models in undergraduate nurse education. *Journal of Clinical Nursing, 26,* 4707–4715. doi: 10.1111/jocn.13822

Revell, S. M., & McCurry, M. K. (2010). Engaging millennial learners: Effectiveness of personal response system technology with nursing students in small and large classrooms. *Journal of Nursing Education, 49*(5), 272–275. http://dx.doi.org/10.3928/01484834-20091217-07

Rodriguez, T., & Lapiz-Bluhm, D. (2018). Community service learning in undergraduate nursing: Impact and insights among students. *Journal of Nursing Practice and Applications & Reviews of Research, 8*(2), 42–49. https://doi.org/10.13178/jnparr.2018.0802.0807

Rundle, S., & Dunn, R. (2008). Building excellence (BE)® BE 2000 research manual 1996–2008. Rochester, NY: Performance Concepts International.

Sedden, M. L., & Clark, K. R. (2016). Motivating students in the 21st century. *Radiologic Technology, 87*(6), 609–614.

Staykova, M. P., Von Stewart, D., & Staykov, D. I. (2017). Back to basics and beyond: Comparing traditional and innovative strategies for teaching in nursing skills laboratories. *Teaching and Learning in Nursing, 12,* 152–157. http://dx.doi.org/10.1016/j.teln.2016.12.001

Tanner, C. (2006). Thinking like a nurse: A research-based model of clinical judgment in nursing. *Journal of Nursing Education, 45*(6), 204–211.

Thompson, B. (2016). The connected classroom: Using digital technology to promote learning. In D. M. Billings & J. A. Halstead (Eds.), *Teaching in nursing: A guide for faculty* (5th ed., pp. 324–341). St. Louis, MO: Elsevier.

Valiee, S., Glorokh, M., Khaledi, S., & Garibi, F. (2016). Nursing students' perspectives on clinical instructors' effective teaching strategies: A descriptive study. *Nurse Education in Practice, 16,* 258–262. https://dx.doi.org/10.1016/j.nepr.2015.09.009

Varagona, L. M., & Hold, J. L. (2019). Nursing students' perceptions of faculty trustworthiness: Thematic analysis of a longitudinal study. *Nurse Education Today, 72,* 27–31. https://doi.org/10.1016/j.nedt.2018.10.008

Wells, M. I., & Dellinger, A. B. (2011). The effect of type of learning environment on perceived learning among graduate nursing students. *Nursing Education Perspectives, 32*(6), 406–410.

Wiggs, C. M. (2010). Collaborative testing: Assessing teamwork and critical thinking behaviors in baccalaureate students. *Nurse Education Today, 31*(3), 279–282. doi:10.1016/j.nedt.2010.10.027.

Yang-Heui, A., & Choi, J. (2019). Incivility experiences in clinical practicum education among nursing students. *Nurse Education Today, 73,* 48–53. https://doi.org/10.1016/j.nedt.2018.11.015

2

Facilitate Learner Development and Socialization

Susan Luparell, PhD, RN, CNE, ANEF

The CNE® Test Plan lists the following for the area of Facilitate Learner Development and Socialization:

Facilitate Learner Development and Socialization

  A. Identify individual learning styles and unique learning needs of learners with these characteristics:
    1. culturally diverse (including international)
    2. English as an additional language
    3. traditional versus nontraditional (i.e., recent high school graduates vs. those in school later)
    4. at risk (e.g., educationally disadvantaged, learning and/or physically challenged, social, and economic issues)
    5. previous nursing education
  B. Provide resources for diverse learners to meet their individual learning needs.
  C. Advise learners in ways that help them meet their professional goals.
  D. Create learning environments that facilitate learners' self-reflection, personal goal setting, and socialization to the role of the nurse.
  E. Foster the development of learners in these areas:
    1. cognitive domain
    2. psychomotor domain
    3. affective domain
  F. Assist learners to engage in thoughtful and constructive self-evaluation and peer evaluation.
  G. Encourage professional development of learners.

According to the National League for Nursing (NLN), competent educators "recognize their responsibility for helping students develop as nurses and integrate the values and behaviors of those who fulfill that role" (NLN, n.d.). Additionally, the American Nurses Association (ANA) Code of Ethics (2015) calls on educators "to ensure that all their graduates possess the knowledge, skills, and moral dispositions that are essential to nursing" (p. 44).

As will be discussed throughout this chapter, to fulfill these expectations, educators must be able to:

- appreciate and attend to the various learning styles of their students
- appreciate and address unique learning needs of an increasingly diverse student body, including nontraditional students, those with disabilities, and those for whom English is an additional language (EAL)
- advise students in a way that fosters both personal and professional development
- create learning environments that facilitate self-reflection, goal-setting, and socialization to the role of nurse

- foster student development in the cognitive, psychomotor, and affective domains
- encourage ongoing professional development

Therefore, this chapter explores the role of faculty in facilitating learner development and socialization from a perspective beyond knowledge acquisition.

Socialization is defined as "the nurturing, acceptance, and integration of a person into the profession of nursing" (Norris, 2017, p. 413), whereby that person comes to identify as a nurse. Professional identity as a nurse is further defined as "a sense of oneself that is influenced by characteristics, norms, and values of the nursing discipline, resulting in an individual thinking, acting, and feeling like a nurse" (Godfrey & Crigger, 2017, p. 379). "Being" a nurse is characterized not only by providing care that meets acceptable practice standards but also by acting ethically and professionally in the broader facets of daily personal and professional life. Further, professional identity formation is a difficult, continuous, and dynamic process during which individuals can be expected to both progress and slip (Godfrey & Crigger, 2017). Educators are instrumental in creating experiences that facilitate professional identity formation and in guiding students to navigate the difficult intrapersonal transitions associated with it.

Societal changes have influenced the manner in which traditional students mature and develop, resulting in delays in reaching full adulthood (Arnett, 2004). Instead, emerging adulthood is now recognized as an important life stage between adolescence and adulthood and spans the years 18 through 29. There are five key features of emerging adults (Arnett, 2004) as noted in Figure 2.1. It is easy to see that faculty may be befuddled by the behaviors of students transitioning into adulthood. One minute students may embrace practice as nurse professionals, while the next minute they may appear unable to take adult responsibility for their learning.

Additionally, for most students, the nursing curriculum represents a discrete portion of a broader college experience. This is a period of intense change, especially for traditional students, and may be accompanied by intense stress and anxiety from multiple sources. Therefore, nurse educators should be familiar with some of the major theoretical perspectives that guide understanding of traditional

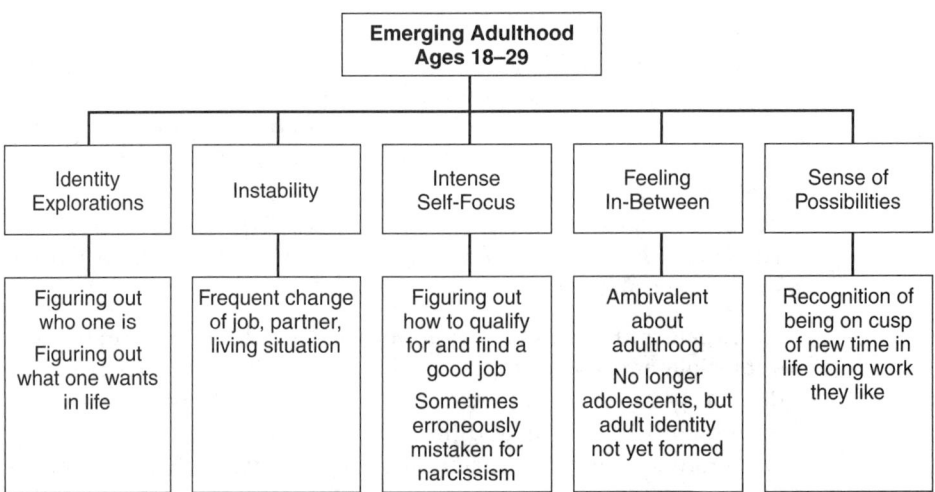

FIGURE 2.1 Features of emerging adulthood.

student development in college. For example, *identity development theories* attempt to explain how college students come to know themselves personally and interpersonally, while *cognitive-structural development theories* attempt to explain how college students develop higher-level thinking and reasoning skills (Broido & Schreiber, 2016). Both of these perspectives are informative to nurse educators seeking to foster learner development on multiple planes. Student affairs professionals are experts in college student development; it is wise to cultivate relationships and conversations with this group to gain additional insights on these perspectives.

FACULTY AS ADVISERS

Faculty often find themselves serving as academic advisers. Tinto (2016) noted that three factors are key in a student's motivation to persist in a curriculum: self-efficacy, a sense of belonging, and perceived value of the curriculum. Advisers are in a position to positively influence each of these (Zarges, Adams, Higgins, & Muhovich, 2018). The role of faculty as academic adviser has not been well studied specific to nursing education, but it exists as a specialty function in higher education and is based on the premise that "educational goals and purposes need to be extended beyond acquiring knowledge to include the development of individual students' capacities for personal empowerment as autonomous intellectual agents" (White, 2015, p. 271).

As noted in Table 2.1, there are various approaches to advising. Each serves a different purpose and each has advantages and disadvantages (He & Hutson, 2016).

Academic advising is meant to aid individual students, but it can take place in small groups or one-on-one, in person or at a distance, synchronously or

Table 2.1

Types of Advising

Type of Advising Approach	Purpose	Sample Tasks

Prescriptive	Information sharing	• Inform student on how to:
		  • choose correct courses
		  • register for courses
		  • file for financial aid
		  • get parking pass
		  • file grievance paperwork

Proactive (intrusive)	Mitigate problems early	• Keep tabs on at-risk student performance. • Assist with plan for time management. • Refer to tutoring services and other learning resources.

Developmental	Holistic personal and professional development	• Assist student to:
		  • identify personal strengths and weaknesses
		  • identify personal and professional goals
		  • consider advantages and disadvantages of potential job offers
		  • problem-solve academic issues

Table 2.2

Desirable Adviser Values and Characteristics

Desirable Values	Desirable Skills and Characteristics
• Caring • Commitment • Empowerment • Inclusivity • Integrity • Professionalism	• Knowledgeable about advising role • Knowledgeable about institutional and college policies, procedures, curriculum, and resources • Good interpersonal skills, including building rapport • Good communication skills • Skills in facilitating problem-solving and goal setting • Acting as student advocate • Organized and timely • Welcoming • Authentic

Data from NACADA: The Global Community for Academic Advising. (2017a). NACADA core values of academic advising. Retrieved from https://www.nacada.ksu.edu/Resources/Pillars/CoreValues.aspx; and NACADA: The Global Community for Academic Advising. (2017b). NACADA academic advising core competencies model. Retrieved from https://www.nacada.ksu.edu/Resources/Pillars/Core Competencies.aspx

asynchronously (White, 2015). Faculty should be welcoming and spend time getting to know the advisee, including personal and professional goals, as well as potential challenges to success, such as financial constraints, learning needs, and personal circumstances that may impact success. The amount and quality of interactions has been shown to influence student satisfaction with advising (DeLaRosby, 2017); thus, faculty advisers should be readily available and approachable. Other desirable adviser characteristics are listed in Table 2.2.

For those wishing to learn more, the National Academic Advising Association (NACADA) is an excellent resource. Lastly, because of their potential impact on student success, faculty are encouraged to evaluate the quality of both individual and program-level academic advising. Important outcomes include student satisfaction, student self-efficacy, and various forms of student success.

Scenario 2.1

A faculty adviser is meeting with a new nursing student for the first time. The student is nervous and has several questions about getting off on the right foot in classes.

Consider: Create a plan for this first session that incorporates aspects of prescriptive as well as developmental advising.

FOSTERING LEARNER DEVELOPMENT IN THREE DOMAINS OF LEARNING

Dr. Benjamin Bloom and his colleagues identified three domains toward which learning activities should be directed and developed taxonomies, or classifications, for each (Anderson & Krathwohl, 2001). Each domain includes a series of developmental levels, or hierarchies, to be achieved, starting with the most basic functions of the domain and moving toward the more complex. The goal of the faculty is to help the student mature and develop in each domain; the nurse educator should plan teaching and learning activities that challenge the student to attain the highest levels of proficiency possible. Educators should be familiar with the domains of learning and their taxonomies, which should be used to guide faculty in (1) developing instructional objectives, (2) choosing teaching and learning strategies, and (3) planning learner assessment (McDonald, 2018).

Cognitive Domain

The cognitive domain addresses learning at six progressively more complex levels of sophistication. At the most basic level, students should be able to *remember* factual information. As a student develops in the cognitive domain, activities should be geared toward increasingly higher-level cognitive function. The student should *understand* the meaning of the information and *apply* it to relevant scenarios. Teachers should guide learners to *analyze* and *evaluate* information. At the highest level of cognitive function, students should be able to *create* new meanings and experiences with the information in hand. It is generally presumed that students move up the hierarchy in a somewhat linear fashion. That is, a student cannot *apply* information on potassium levels if the student does not first *understand* what potassium regulates and what the normal levels are.

To best foster student development, the faculty must be cognizant of the ultimate goal and create activities that promote advancement up the hierarchy of cognitive learning. For example, flash cards may help students learn important medical terms, but matching alone limits the student to the recall level of proficiency and provides little stimulus for developing more complex understanding. On the other hand, case studies require the student to analyze information in the context of the study. Alternatively, development of a concept map linking the relationship between immune function, sleep, and nutrition would require a student to understand the most important concepts of each and create a product that visually portrays the linkages.

Psychomotor Domain

It is important to patients that the nurse safely and competently carries out skills. The psychomotor domain addresses the development of motor skills; complexity of achievement ranges from observing and imitating to fine-tuning and adapting to unique situations. For example, at higher levels of psychomotor function, a student would be able to adapt a skill based on the specific type of equipment available or based on a patient's unique needs. As a general rule, frequent repetition is a prerequisite of skills proficiency. Faculty should consider factoring in opportunities for ongoing practice during course and curriculum planning.

Affective Domain

The affective domain is associated with attitudes, beliefs, values, and personal insight, and is especially important for strong professional identity development (Valiga, 2014). As with the other domains, the affective domain is also associated with increasing level of achievement, ranging from simple acknowledgment of a belief or value to its full embodiment demonstrated by how one lives on a daily basis, even when not at work (Godfrey & Crigger, 2017; Valiga, 2014). To effectively address the affective domain, the nurse educator must develop teaching strategies and learning activities that stimulate an emotional response or cause a student to reconsider values and beliefs. For example, a class debate exposing two sides of an ethical issue may cause intrapersonal conflict resulting in critical introspection about what one believes and why.

LEARNING STYLES

It is commonly understood that learners possess various learning styles. That is, each learner has a preferred method of taking in and making sense of information. Ideally, educators tap into the unique learning styles of their students to maximize students' learning but also to increase the overall value of the educational experience. Although there are numerous theories and frameworks available to guide educators' planning, two common models are discussed in this chapter. Additional information on learning theories may be found in Chapter 1.

Kolb's Experiential Learning Theory (ELT) and Kolb's Learning Styles

One of the most common frameworks seen in the higher education and nursing literature is Kolb's Experiential Learning Theory (ELT), which also serves as the basis for understanding learning styles associated with it. Several propositions serve as the foundation for the ELT. Key among these are as follows:

- New learning is really the relearning, rethinking, and refining of one's old ideas.
- Learning is driven by conflict among competing ideas, requiring the learner to move back and forth between reflecting and acting, as well as feeling and thinking.
- Learning is a process and the educator should provide feedback about the effectiveness of the learner's efforts (Kolb & Kolb, 2005).

Thus, according to the ELT, educators should focus not only on the content of the learning but also on the processes of learning, including how the students go about learning.

Kolb's ELT suggests that the learning process is cyclical and that, although a learner may enter the process at any stage, eventually the learner must progress through all. A typical process includes the learner having a concrete experience, upon which the learner reflects deeply. Such reflection leads to analysis of old experiences and drawing of new conclusions. These are then applied in new situations and result in new experiences that restart the cycle (McLeod, 2017). Instructors who espouse the ELT create learning experiences that adeptly lead learners through each of these stages. That is, they employ teaching strategies that permit students to consider how new content fits contextually with their past experiences and vice versa, and how it can be applied to new experiences.

Additionally, it is thought that superimposed on this cyclical process lie two dissecting continuums that represent how learners prefer to receive and process information. One continuum captures learner preference for perceiving information, while the other captures learner preference for processing that information. An individual will take in information in either a highly active manner or in a more reflective manner. Additionally, an individual will tend to process that information very concretely, very abstractly, or somewhere in between. Helpful graphic depictions of the experiential learning cycle and these two continuums may be viewed at https://www.simplypsychology.org/learning-kolb.html. Although students may have patterns and preferences for certain learning styles over others, these styles should be considered dynamic, rather than fixed, traits (Kolb & Kolb, 2005; McLeod, 2017). A learning styles inventory is available to assess where students may presently fall on these continuums and, more recently, it has been suggested that nine learning styles may be differentiated (Kolb & Kolb, 2012). Astute faculty should design learning activities that acknowledge these various preferences. Table 2.3 outlines teaching

Table 2.3

Potential Teaching Strategies for Kolb's Learning Styles

	Characteristics	Teaching Strategies
Divergers	• Prefer to watch and gather information • Imaginative • Good at viewing situations from different perspectives • Good at brainstorming	• Plan group activities. • Provide opportunities for reflection. • Provide opportunities for creative problem-solving.
Assimilators	• Highly logical and organized • Less focused on people than on ideas • Enjoy reading and lectures	• Provide clear explanations and rationale. • Allow time to think and organize content. • Include theoretical perspectives.
Convergers	• Prefer technical tasks and finding practical solutions • Less concerned with interpersonal aspects	• Plan practical problem-solving activities. • Allow experimentation. • Provide simulation.
Accommodators	• Rely on intuition over logic • Tend to rely on others for information	• Plan practical problem-solving.

Data from McLeod, S. A. (2017). Kolb's learning styles and experiential learning cycle. Retrieved from https://www.simplypsychology.org/learning-kolb.html

strategies for this purpose. However, students should also be guided to engage in learning using means that may be inconsistent with their usual preferences.

Scenario 2.2

A novice nurse educator attends a conference where the nurse educator learns about the need to address various learning styles in the classroom and sets a professional goal to be intentional about doing so. In an upcoming class, the nurse educator wants students to learn the signs and symptoms of congestive heart failure as well as key nursing interventions. The nurse educator goes about planning based on new knowledge of learning styles.

Consider:
1. Identify one teaching strategy that would address each of the Kolb learning styles.
2. Take a concept from a course you teach and draft an instructional plan for moving a learner from a concrete experience to abstract conceptualization.

IDENTIFY UNIQUE NEEDS OF DIVERSE LEARNERS

The nursing student body is increasingly diverse, with students of all ages in our classrooms as well as increasing numbers of men and nonbinary individuals, people of various races and ethnicities, those of different sexual orientations, and those from various socioeconomic backgrounds. Nursing classrooms remain less diverse than college campuses in general, but small changes have become evident over time. For example, Black students comprise 12.2 percent of nursing students, Hispanic students 8.1 percent, and Asian or Pacific Islander students 5.9 percent, increases of 2.8 percent, 4.6 percent, and 1.9 percent, respectively, from 1995 (NLN, 2014). Men, depending on type of nursing program, comprise 9 percent to 15 percent of students (NLN, 2014). Students over the age of 30 years comprise 42 percent of ADN students, 37 percent of LPN students, 30 percent of diploma students, and 18 percent of BSN students (NLN, 2014). No data on student numbers specific to nursing are available, but there are estimates of close to one million LGBTQ (lesbian, gay, bisexual, transgender, transsexual, queer) college students across college campuses (Tramell, 2014). Much work remains to be done to ensure that the nursing profession reflects the population it serves. Both the NLN and the American Association of Colleges of Nursing (AACN) periodically collect demographic data on both students and faculty. Faculty should remain abreast of the demographic characteristics of their unique student body. In this section, we examine some of the key considerations, unique learning styles, and needs related to the increasingly diverse student body.

Age Diversity

Traditional students are those who enter college immediately or soon after the completion of high school, making them relatively young. However, students and faculty in any nursing classroom may represent multiple generations, cohorts of individuals born in roughly the same time frame who have similar experiences and frames of reference. Thus, they tend to share values, attitudes, expectations, and motivational stimuli. To decrease conflict in the classroom and meet the needs of various age groups, faculty must understand the attitudes and values associated with the various generations while at the same time avoiding broad sweeping generalizations. To be effective as educators, teaching and communication should seek to leverage all of the generational preferences, as depicted in Table 2.4.

Table 2.4

Generational Characteristics

Generation	Common Characteristics
Baby Boomers (1945–1964)	• Strong work ethic • Value personal communication • Value career over personal life
Generation X (1965–1979)	• Independent • Intolerant of bureaucracy • Family focused; seek balance • Seek rewards based on individual performance
Millennials (1980–1994)	• Highly socialized • Technologically savvy • Multitaskers • See education as a means to an end • Value personal life over career
Generation Z (after 1995)	• Known characteristics still evolving • Technological savants • Communicate almost exclusively via social media • Appreciate virtual connectedness • Connected at all times • Little tolerance for poor connectivity

Data from Elliott-Yeary, S. (2017). The five generations in the workplace. Retrieved from https://www.generationalguru.com/single-post/2017/06/13/The-Five-Generations-in-the-Workplace

Generation Z students, born after 1995, have recently begun entering college classrooms and display different characteristics than their Millennial predecessors. These students have multiple devices and screens at their disposal and are connected to technology over 10 hours a day (Kleinschmit, 2019). Although our understanding of their general characteristics is still unfolding, these students may need additional role modeling of interpersonal communication necessary for nursing.

There are additional unique groups of students who may have specific learning needs. There are multiple organizations and journals that focus on understanding and serving the diverse student body. Both the National Association of Student Affairs Professionals (NASAP) and the National Association of Student Personnel Administrators (NASPA) specialize in issues related to student affairs. Additionally, many colleges and universities now have Offices of Diversity and Inclusion that can provide valuable insights and resources to faculty hoping to better understand and meet the needs of unique student groups. Table 2.5 captures some of these groups and their unique learning needs. An expanded discussion of each follows.

Table 2.5

Unique Learner Needs

	Unique Needs	Strategies
English as an Additional Language students (EAL)	• Assistance with time management • Assistance with language and medical terminology • Assistance with cultural assimilation	• Permit audiotaping of classes. • Facilitate time management and scheduling. • Show value for EAL student's native culture and language. • Allow sufficient time for group work and student participation. • Demonstrate patience. • Team with students of program's native language. • Supply tutors/translators as needed. • Facilitate communication with staff and patients.
Ethnic and culturally diverse students	• Assistance assimilating with predominant culture • May experience racism or prejudice • May also be EAL students	• Promote inclusion and respect. • Address episodes of intolerance.
Post 9/11 veterans	• May have physical or psychological comorbidities	• Be sensitive to patient care situations that may expose previous trauma.
Students with disabilities	• May experience stigma or bias • Unique physical, emotional, or cognitive needs related to the disability	• Promote inclusion and respect among students and in exams and assignments. • Refer to Office of Disability Services for formal assessment and determination of accommodations. • Consistently implement required accommodations. • Be sensitive to struggles encountered based on the disability. • Hold to same academic standards as other students.
LBGTQ students	• May or many not wish to be publicly out • Often experience stigma, bias, prejudice, or violence	• Promote inclusion and respect among students and in exams and assignments. • Take care not to out an individual. • If out, use preferred pronouns.

ETHNIC AND CULTURAL DIVERSITY

Although on the increase, the makeup of minorities in nursing programs is not equivalent to the minority representation among all US college students. Culture is a representation of values, habits, and beliefs acquired over time because of membership within a group. It is important to remember that culture is not solely tied to ethnicity and that all individuals belong to multiple groups. Increasingly, nurse educators see students who are first-generation college students or who hail from various socioeconomic backgrounds, family structures, or regions of the country. Whether students are from a rural or urban area will influence their particular approach to learning. Faculty must assess the unique influences of culture on student learning needs and plan teaching accordingly.

EAL Students

Students for whom English is an additional language (EAL), also sometimes referred to as English-language learners (ELLs), represent a further subset of the minority student population. These students are bilingual or multilingual and generally are international or immigrant learners (Olson, 2012). However, faculty should also bear in mind that a student may appear to be English speaking, even having been born in the United States, but may have been raised in a home where the primary language is not English. These students may ostensibly speak English quite well but may actually think and process ideas in an alternative language, which may manifest itself in the form of subtle communication challenges or test-taking difficulties.

Historically, EAL students experience unique challenges in nursing school, most of which stem from language difficulties. For instance, EAL students may have a difficult time understanding medical terminology or communicating with patients and staff. Subsequently, they have higher attrition rates than native speakers and collectively lower NCLEX® pass rates (Olson, 2012). Research has shown that EAL students benefit from working on teams with native English speakers (or the native language of the program). Additionally, it may prove helpful for EAL students to audiotape class sessions and be provided copies of class handouts. Having EAL students perform role-playing activities in which they interact with patients and staff may further facilitate communication skills and relieve their anxiety (Olson, 2012).

Not all challenges faced by EAL students are related to language. International or immigrant students may experience significant conflicts between their own cultural background and the American educational and health care systems (Olson, 2012). Additionally, EAL students may find themselves victims of racism and other stereotyping by fellow students, faculty, agency staff, and patients. To minimize barriers based on culture, faculty should work to create a climate of openness, value, and respect, and allow adequate time for class activities. They should also use care not to conflate language difficulties with lack of intellectual ability.

Gender Diversity

Men may have unique student experiences, especially when it comes to providing care for women. During obstetric clinical experiences, for example, laboring women or their partners may feel uncomfortable with a male student, or some men may have concerns about being falsely accused of improprieties when delivering perineal or other intimate care to a woman.

Traditional versus Nontraditional Learners

Although increasingly diverse, traditional learners typically are those who are entering a prelicensure nursing program almost immediately following high school. They tend to have limited work and life experience, and usually do not have family responsibilities. The term *nontraditional learner* refers to a student who may (1) be older, (2) have significant work experience (but no formal higher education), (3) be the first to attend college in the family, (4) have full- or part-time employment, or (5) have a spouse and/or children. Nontraditional students are known to have different life stressors than their traditional counterparts, but they may lack peers among their classmates to whom they can turn for support. Therefore, educators should be vigilant in assessing the well-being of these students and be knowledgeable about resources available to assist them.

It has long been posited that adult learners approach education differently than traditional students; educators should be cognizant of these differences. For example, adult learners tend to be motivated by a need to know content that they recognize as relevant to help them meet their goals. They also tend to be more self-directed and expect to have an active role in their learning, which is greatly informed by their previous life experiences. All of these characteristics should be valued by faculty (Chen, 2014).

Students with Previous Education

There has been a burgeoning of accelerated nursing programs in recent years into which are enrolled adult students who have already obtained college degrees in another field. These students choose to come into nursing for a variety of reasons, including a desire to follow through on a previous interest or acquire stable employment. They tend to have diverse characteristics, most notably in terms of background and experiences, and many have multiple responsibilities outside of school (Siler, DeBasio, & Roberts, 2008). Accelerated students may also experience unique financial constraints since accelerated programs are more time-intensive than traditional programs.

Evidence suggests that second-degree students, as adult learners, desire different teaching approaches for success. However, accelerated nursing students may face multiple barriers to learning. These include an unsupportive environment for learning, ineffective teaching methods, and stress. Based on the characteristics of this group of learners, strategies that may facilitate student success include those that involve experiential learning, self-directed learning, and the social-cognitive theory of learning (Chen, 2014). In particular, faculty should consider employing teaching strategies that allow students to assimilate their new nursing knowledge with previous experiences.

Students with Disabilities

A disabled person has physical or mental impairment that substantially limits one or more major life activities, which include "seeing, hearing, eating, smelling, sleeping, breathing, walking, speaking, bowel and bladder control, learning, reading, writing, spelling, concentrating, thinking, communicating, perceiving and other neurologic functions, working, performing self care and other manual tasks" (Southern Regional Education Board [SREB], n.d.). Students with visible or invisible disabilities are protected by federal law under the Americans with Disabilities Act (ADA) of 1990 and the ADA Amendment Act of 2008, which guarantee that persons who are otherwise qualified for admission cannot be denied access based on disability alone, nor can they be otherwise discriminated against. Students must self-disclose a disability to the educational institution, which is then responsible for providing reasonable accommodations to assist the student to successfully meet program outcomes (SREB, n.d.). Individual faculty should not determine which accommodations are needed. Rather, this assessment is performed by the disability services officer—faculty should consult with the officer to seek additional guidance when working with students.

At-Risk Students

Students who are the first in their family to attend college may encounter unique challenges because they lack access to parents or siblings who have experienced higher education. For example, they may be unfamiliar with common vocabulary used in higher education, processes for class enrollment, procedures for seeking housing, procedures for seeking financial aid, and resources available to facilitate success. According to the US Department of Education (Redford & Hoyer, 2017), first-generation students tend to be from lower socioeconomic households and over half are from minority households. They are more likely to drop out owing to financial constraints (Redford & Hoyer, 2017). They tend to have higher attrition rates and lower grade point averages. The role of the academic adviser is key.

Some students may be economically disadvantaged, either because they come from a lower socioeconomic household, have multiple financial responsibilities outside of school, or are independently responsible for their education. Faculty should be aware of the many expenses associated with school, including textbook prices, tuition and housing, and extraneous fees and expenses, such as required travel for clinical experiences. Keeping those in mind, faculty should avoid requiring activities that add unnecessary or unplanned costs.

Scenario 2.3

On the first day of class, a student discloses to a faculty member that the student has a documented learning disability and requires accommodations.

Consider: What steps should the faculty member take in managing this student?

Scenario 2.4

A student for whom English is an additional language has received a failing score on the first exam of the course. The student is tearful and is considering dropping out of the curriculum.

Consider: How might an instructor intervene to assist this student?

FACILITATING CRITICAL THINKING AND REFLECTIVE PRACTICE

The ability to reflect on one's actions in a given set of circumstances is an important component of identify formation. As described in the hallmark Carnegie study on nursing education (Benner, Sutphen, Leonard, & Day, 2010), faculty should aspire to teach for salience, coaching students to reflect on experiences to determine the most important features. In doing so, students begin to learn to discern the relevant from the irrelevant. Consistent with experiential learning theory, reflection plays an important role in a student's growth.

To enhance reflection, faculty need to guide students to think deeply by using high-level questions that require students to more fully analyze a situation, consider how they determined which actions to take or not to take, and to expose their decision-making (Oermann, Shellenbarger, & Gaberson, 2018). Activities such as group discussions, clinical conferences, and journaling can provide opportunities for reflection on practice. Examples of high-level guiding questions designed to foster deep thinking and clinical reasoning include:

- "I see you decided to forego your assessment to let the patient sleep a bit longer. What information did you have in determining that it was okay to do so? What would have made you decide to wake him up?"
- "I see you administered the patient's antihypertensive medication. What helped you determine that it was appropriate to go ahead and give it? Is there anything that could have occurred that would have made you hold it instead?"

While these types of questions are particularly useful when students have made errors in judgment, they are also important for guiding students to reflect on appropriate practice. In this way, students can use those experiences to inform their learning as well.

The evidence on simulation as a strategy to improve critical thinking is still evolving but is promising. A large umbrella systematic review found that simulation "benefited nursing students in terms of knowledge acquisition and critical thinking; it increased standardized critical thinking test scores, enhanced students' scores on knowledge and skills exams, and created a learning environment that contributed to greater knowledge, skills, safety, and students' confidence" (Cant & Cooper, 2017, p. 65). Faculty who incorporate simulation into their courses should be well versed on simulation best practices, especially as they relate to developing, implementing, and debriefing scenarios. Other teaching strategies, such as the use of unfolding cases (Hong & Yu, 2017) and concept mapping (Yue, Zhang, Zhang, & Jin, 2017), may also be useful in promoting critical thinking.

ASSISTING LEARNERS TO ENGAGE IN CONSTRUCTIVE EVALUATION OF SELF AND OTHERS

In addition to facilitating learner development in the cognitive and psychomotor domains of learning, faculty are also tasked to help foster affective learning as a part of professional identity formation, in which students internalize the values of the profession. Consistent with Kolb's Experiential Learning Theory discussed earlier in this chapter, feedback is a critical component of the learning process. Likewise, an important component of professional maturity is the ability to thoughtfully and constructively analyze performance and provide feedback to facilitate improvement. This process must occur at both the individual and team levels. To enhance the learner's ability to engage in self-evaluation, faculty should include opportunities for students to do so.

Providing realistic and honest feedback while avoiding being intentionally hurtful is a skill that will be useful to students in the working world. Faculty should incorporate opportunities for students to learn this skill and should frequently remind students of the importance that honest self-appraisal plays in role development. Examples include self-reflection journals and guided introspection. Additionally, faculty should role model the proper way to provide constructive feedback in their dealings with students. A trusting relationship is essential in providing feedback. Faculty should remind students often that the motive for sharing constructive feedback is to ultimately see the student succeed and flourish in the nursing role. Activities in which students must provide feedback to their peers may also be useful in enhancing skills.

As might be expected, there is great variation in the amount and type of feedback that individual students desire or require; faculty should be as responsive as possible to these needs. Oermann et al. (2018) identified additional key principles to guide delivery of constructive feedback. These include:

- Deliver feedback in a way that is specific and precisely identifies the behavior that needs to be corrected.
- Deliver feedback in a timely manner, when details of the problematic behavior are more likely to be remembered accurately by both student and teacher.
- Deliver feedback incorporating verbal and visual cues to help the student understand what the problematic behavior entailed and what correct behavior would look like.
- Feedback should be diagnostic in nature, so that students can learn where deficiencies in practice exist and work to alleviate them.

Scenario 2.5

During a clinical experience in an acute care course, a staff nurse informs the instructor that the staff nurse witnessed the student interact unprofessionally with one of the nursing assistants. The student was reported to have refused to assist the aide with ambulating a patient, saying to the aide, "That's your job, not mine" before leaving to go on break.

Consider:
1. What principles should guide the instructor's feedback to this student?
2. Script out the beginning of the conversation in which feedback about this situation is delivered to the student.

ENCOURAGE PROFESSIONAL DEVELOPMENT AND SOCIALIZATION TO THE ROLE

Faculty are in a prime position to influence students' attitudes about professional organizations and lifelong learning. Role modeling, both positive and negative, has been shown to have a powerful impact on students (Felstead & Springett, 2016). Faculty can role model ongoing professional development in many ways, including talking about their own professional activities. Alternatively, faculty might interrupt class when a question is asked for which the answer is not known and have the whole group access resources to answer the question. Faculty can also encourage students to attend local conferences as a value-added part of a course; even better, faculty can attend a conference with students and demonstrate networking and ongoing learning.

Incivility, horizontal violence, and nurse bullying are important topics in health care and have been well-documented. Contemporary evidence suggests that incivility is linked to nurses' decreased job satisfaction and increased patient harm (Dang, Bae, Karlowicz, & Kim, 2016; Institute for Safe Medication Practices, 2013). Therefore, in terms of socialization, the ethical imperative to graduate students who improve the work environment rather than detract from it is significant. Unfortunately, evidence suggests that some poorly behaving students continue that behavior post-licensure (Luparell & Frisbee, 2019). To best facilitate development of professional comportment, especially as it relates to interpersonal interactions in the profession, faculty should make civility in their classrooms a priority. Students need clear delineation of behavioral expectations and why these expectations are important to patient safety. Additionally, faculty themselves, as role models of the profession, must embrace civility in their interactions with students and each other.

SUMMARY

Although novice faculty may initially perceive their primary role to be one of sharing knowledge and expertise with students, most seasoned faculty would suggest that the role is both much more complex and much more subtle. Faculty have profound influence over student development on many levels. For students to maximize their potential, the learning environment must be one in which students perceive that they are free to explore ideas and try new things without undue persecution. To best facilitate learning, faculty are charged with understanding their students both collectively and as individuals. Only after gaining such insight can faculty set about meeting student learning needs.

Practice Test Questions

1. Assisting a student to do which of the following would be evident of intrusive advising?
   A. Choosing appropriate course sequencing
   B. Identifying deadlines for scholarship application
   C. Considering career goals when job seeking
   D. Accessing the writing center after receiving a poor grade on a paper

2. To facilitate learning in EAL students, the instructor should consider which of the following?
   A. Providing an in-class translator for the student
   B. Pairing the student with others who speak the same native language
   C. Providing a reference sheet explaining common medical terms and axioms
   D. Giving timed in-class assignments

3. Which of the following is true regarding professional identity formation?
   A. It requires a person to internalize the values and behaviors of the nursing profession.
   B. It is a process whereby external rules are imposed on the new nurse.
   C. The longer one is in school, the more likely that person will achieve professional identity.
   D. The tendency to develop as a nurse professional is innate and cannot be developed.

4. A student nearly makes a serious medication error in the clinical setting after failing to double-check the dose. The student is visibly shaken after realizing the near miss. In providing feedback about this incident to the student, how should the instructor proceed?
   A. Immediately discuss what almost happened while still at the patient's bedside.
   B. Discuss the incident in clinical conference so that other students can also learn from the mistake.
   C. Discuss the incident more fully the following week, after the student has a chance to remediate the performance.
   D. Discuss the incident privately with the student that same day.

5. Which of the following is consistent with emerging adulthood?
   A. Changing majors multiple times in the first two years of college
   B. Becoming angry at the instructor when a poor grade is received on an assignment
   C. Privately volunteering for an event in order to contribute to a greater good
   D. Establishing a loving, intimate relationship with someone

6. An instructor has already taught concepts of intravenous therapy for dehydration. In attempting to move learners to the active experimentation stage of learning, the instructor should have students do which of the following?
   A. Consider how intravenous therapy is used to manage postoperative fluid shifts.
   B. Evaluate urine output in patients receiving intravenous therapy.

C. Make a list of conditions in which intravenous therapy would be contraindicated.

D. Memorize the osmolality of various intravenous fluids.

7. Which of the following would likely appeal to learners who demonstrate the diverging learning style?
   A. Developing a case study that highlights key class concepts
   B. Working in groups to create a care plan based on a case study
   C. Watching a film in class followed by discussion on how the main protagonist overcame challenges
   D. Having students create a concept map linking the main themes of the class session

8. Which of the following would likely appeal to learners who demonstrate the converging learning style?
   A. Allowing students to self-determine an appropriate way to perform a procedure as long as key guidelines for safety are followed
   B. Giving a step-by-step set of instructions for performing a procedure
   C. Showing a skills video in class and having students return demonstrate a procedure
   D. Having students recite the steps of a procedure and describe how to perform it

9. Which is the most important strategy for the nurse educator to implement when preparing to teach a group of adult learners?
   A. Develop learning experiences that build on previous experiences and learning.
   B. Provide highly structured learning activities that limit individualization of learning.
   C. Avoid the use of teaching strategies that foster reflective practice.
   D. Minimize learner participation in identifying their learning needs.

10. The nursing instructor expects the students in a pathophysiology course to be able to correlate the physiological changes experienced by complex medical patients with their clinical manifestations and complications. Which strategy should the instructor choose to best facilitate this analysis?
    A. Concept mapping
    B. Algorithms
    C. One-minute paper
    D. Clinical simulation

11. Which learning outcome represents the highest achievement in the cognitive domain?
    A. Describe the effect of loop diuretics on serum potassium levels.
    B. Evaluate the efficacy of incentive spirometry to a patient's oxygenation.
    C. Differentiate among calcium channel blockers and ACE inhibitors.
    D. Develop a plan of care for a patient with bacterial pneumonia.

12. A fourth-year baccalaureate nursing student is having trouble inserting intravenous catheters and is not demonstrating aseptic technique. This skill was previously taught in the Fundamentals course. What action should the instructor initiate to best rectify this situation?
    A. Fail the student in the course for not mastering this skill.
    B. Assign a short paper on how to maintain aseptic technique during catheterization.
    C. Refer the student to the nursing lab instructor for coaching and remedial practice.
    D. Have the student reflect on strengths and weaknesses in the clinical area in the weekly journal.

13. A new nurse educator is attempting to address various learning styles when delivering didactic contact. What is the most important concept that will facilitate this endeavor?
    A. Develop at least one classroom activity that meets the needs of each representative learning style.
    B. Assign group classroom activities in which each group is composed of students with different learning styles.
    C. Communicate to students that completion of classroom activities will provide the necessary tools for success.
    D. Provide classroom activities that encourage faculty-student interaction.

14. Which student learning outcome best represents the affective domain of learning?
    A. Develop basic plans of care using the nursing process for patients with common alterations in health status.
    B. Conduct an initial physical assessment of a patient with common health-related interference in functional health patterns.
    C. Respond to aspects of sociocultural influences that impact the health of families.
    D. Identify and apply relevant principles of pathophysiology related to alterations in metabolism.

15. Which student support intervention would be most beneficial to facilitate learning for EAL students?
    A. Provide individual tutoring sessions, especially for the EAL students.
    B. Require EAL students to take additional English language classes.
    C. Require EAL students to complete assignments both in writing and orally.
    D. Plan team-based learning strategies that partner EAL and native English speakers.

16. The instructor who draws on experiential learning theory would use which of the following principles in course planning?
    A. How students go about learning requires as much attention as what they are learning.
    B. Students need to share common experiences to form a sense of community.
    C. Students need to shed their understanding of previous life experiences.
    D. New modes of learning will be required to teach students with diverse backgrounds.

17. What is the primary rationale underpinning the faculty's responsibility to ensure appropriate student behavior and ethical comportment?
A. Maintain control of the classroom
B. Preserve the image of the profession
C. Facilitate learning
D. Ensure patient safety

18. Which behavior to assist students represents developmental advising?
A. Submit application materials for the licensure exam.
B. Reflect on factors that may have impacted test performance.
C. Register early for required classes.
D. Apply for appropriate scholarship opportunities.

19. Which statement is true regarding the Americans with Disabilities Act?
A. The faculty member is responsible for identifying a student's disability and providing accommodations.
B. Students with disabilities must be able to perform the essential functions of the nursing student role.
C. A school must expend all efforts to ensure that accommodations are provided.
D. Students with disabilities are to be assessed using a different set of criteria from other students.

20. Which student learning outcome best represents the affective domain of learning?
A. Develop basic plans of care using the nursing process for patients with common alterations in health status.
B. Conduct an initial physical assessment of a patient with common health-related interference in functional health patterns.
C. Respond to aspects of sociocultural influences that impact the health of families.
D. Identify and apply relevant principles of pathophysiology related to alterations in metabolism.

References

American Nurses Association. (2015). *Code of ethics for nurses with interpretive statements*. Washington, DC: American Nurses Publishing.

Anderson, L. W., & Krathwohl, D. R. (Eds.). (2001). A taxonomy for learning, teaching and assessing: A revision of Bloom's Taxonomy of educational objectives: Complete edition, New York, NY: Longman.

Arnett, J. J. (2004). *Emerging adulthood: The winding road from the late teens through the twenties*. New York, NY: Oxford University Press.

Benner, P., Sutphen, M., Leonard, V., & Day, L. (2010). *Educating nurses: A call for radical transformation*. San Francisco, CA: Jossey-Bass.

Broido, E. M., & Schreiber, B. (2016). Promoting student learning and development. *New Directions for Higher Education*, 2016(175), 65–74. doi:10.1002/he.20200

Cant, R. P., & Cooper, S. J. (2017). Use of simulation-based learning in undergraduate nurse education: An umbrella systematic review. *Nurse Education Today*, 49, 63–71. doi:10.1016/j.nedt.2016.11.015

Chen, J. C. (2014). Teaching nontraditional adult students: adult learning theories in practice. *Teaching in Higher Education*, 19(4), 406–418. https://doi.org/10.1080/13562517.2013.860101

Dang, D., Bae, S.-H., Karlowicz, K. A., & Kim, M. T. (2016). Do clinician disruptive behaviors make an unsafe environment for patients? *Journal of Nursing Care Quality*, 31(2), 115–123. doi:10.1097/ncq.0000000000000150

DeLaRosby, H. R. (2017). Student characteristics and collegiate environments that contribute to the overall satisfaction with academic advising among college students. *Journal of College Student Retention: Research, Theory & Practice*, 19(2), 145–160. doi: https://doi.org/10.1353/jge.2015.0024

Elliott-Yeary, S. (2017). The five generations in the workplace. Retrieved from https://www.generationalguru.com/single-post/2017/06/13/The-Five-Generations-in-the-Workplace

Felstead, I. S., & Springett, K. (2016). An exploration of role model influence on adult nursing students' professional development: A phenomenological research study. *Nurse Education Today, 37*, 66–70. doi:https://doi.org/10.1016/j.nedt.2015.11.014

Godfrey, N., & Crigger, N. (2017). Professional identity. In J. F. Giddens (Ed.), *Concepts for nursing practice* (2nd ed., pp. 379–386). St. Louis, MO: Elsevier.

He, Y., & Hutson, B. (2016). Appreciative assessment in academic advising. *Review of Higher Education, 39*(2), 213–240. doi: 10.1353/rhe.2016.0003

Hong, S., & Yu, P. (2017). Comparison of the effectiveness of two styles of case-based learning implemented in lectures for developing nursing students' critical thinking ability: A randomized controlled trial. *International Journal of Nursing Studies, 68*, 16–24. doi:10.1016/j.ijnurstu.2016.12.008

Institute for Safe Medication Practices (ISMP). (2013). Unresolved disrespectful behavior in healthcare: Practitioners speak up (again), Part 1. *ISMP Safety Alert Newsletter/Nurse Advise-ERR, 11*(10), 1–4.

Kleinschmit, M. (2019). Generation Z characteristics: 5 infographics on the Gen Z lifestyle. Retrieved from https://www.visioncritical.com/blog/generation-z-infographics

Kolb, A. Y., & Kolb, D. A. (2005). Learning styles and learning spaces: Enhancing experiential learning in higher education. *Academy of Management Learning and Education, 4*(2), 193–212.

Kolb, A. Y., & Kolb, D. A. (2012) Experiential learning spaces. In N. M Seel (Ed.), *Encyclopedia of the sciences of learning*. Boston, MA: Springer. doi: https://doi.org/10.1007/978-1-4419-1428-6

Luparell, S., & Frisbee, K. (2019). Do uncivil nursing students become uncivil nurses? A national survey of faculty perceptions. *Nursing Education Perspectives, 49*(6), 322–327.

McDonald, M. (2018). *The nurse educator's guide to assessing learning outcomes* (4th ed.). Burlington, MA: Jones & Bartlett.

McLeod, S. A. (2017). Kolb's learning styles and experiential learning cycle. Retrieved from https://www.simplypsychology.org/learning-kolb.html

NACADA: The Global Community for Academic Advising. (2017a). NACADA core values of academic advising. Retrieved from https://www.nacada.ksu.edu/Resources/Pillars/CoreValues.aspx

NACADA: The Global Community for Academic Advising. (2017b). NACADA academic advising core competencies model. Retrieved from https://www.nacada.ksu.edu/Resources/Pillars/CoreCompetencies.aspx

National League for Nursing. (n.d.) Nurse educator core competency. Retrieved from http://www.nln.org/professional-development-programs/competencies-for-nursing-education/nurse-educator-core-competency

National League for Nursing. (2014). Nursing student demographics. Retrieved from http://www.nln.org/newsroom/nursing-education-statistics/nursing-student-demographics

Norris, T. M. (2017). Making the transition from student to professional nurse. In B. Cherry & S. R. Jacob (Eds.), *Contemporary nursing: Issues, trends, and management* (pp. 413–433). St. Louis, MO: Elsevier.

Oermann, M. H., Shellenbarger, T., & Gaberson, K. B. (2018). *Clinical teaching strategies in nursing* (5th ed.). New York, NY: Springer.

Olson, M. (2012). English-as-a-second language (ESL) nursing student success: A critical review of the literature. *Journal of Cultural Diversity, 19*(1), 26–32.

Redford, J., & Mulvaney Hoyer, K. U.S. Department of Education/National Center for Education Statistics (2017). First-generation and continuing-generation college students: A comparison of high school and postsecondary experiences. Retrieved from https://nces.ed.gov/pubs2018/2018009.pdf

Scheckel, M. (2020). Designing courses and learning experiences. In D. M. Billings & J. A. Halstead (Eds.), *Teaching in nursing: A guide for faculty* (6th ed., pp. 181–201). St. Louis, MO: Elsevier.

Siler, B., DeBasio, N., & Roberts, K. (2008). Profile of non-nurse college graduates enrolled in accelerated baccalaureate curricula: Results of a national study. *Nursing Education Perspectives, 29*(6), 336–341.

Southern Regional Education Board. (n.d.) The Americans with Disabilities Act: Implications for nursing education. Retrieved from https://www.sreb.org/publication/americans-disabilities-act

Tinto, V. (2016). From retention to persistence. *Inside Higher Ed.* Retrieved from https://www.insidehighered.com/views/2016/09/26/how-improve-student-persistence-and-completion-essay

Tramell, J. B. (2014). LGBT challenges in higher education: 5 core principles for success. *Trusteeship Magazine, 22*(3). Retrieved from https://agb.org/trusteeship-article/lgbt-challenges-in-higher-education-today-5-core-principles-for-success/

Valiga, T. M. (2014). Attending to affective domain learning: Essential to prepare the kind of graduates the public needs. *Journal of Nursing Education, 53*(5), 247.

White, E. R. (2015). Academic advising in higher education. *JGE: The Journal of General Education, 64*(4), 263–277. https://doi-org.proxybz.lib.montana.edu:3443/10.1353/jge.2015.0024

Yue, M., Zhang, M., Zhang, C., & Jin, C. (2017). The effectiveness of concept mapping on development of critical thinking in nursing education: A systematic review and meta-analysis. *Nurse Education Today, 52*, 87–94. doi:http://dx.doi.org/10.1016/j.nedt.2017.02.018

Zarges, K. M., Adams, T. A., Higgins, E. M., & Muhovich, N. (2018). Assessing the impact of academic advising: Current issues and future trends. *New Directions for Higher Education, 2018*(184), 47–57. doi: 10.1002/he.20302

Use Assessment and Evaluation Strategies

Gail Baumlein, PhD, MSN, RN, CNE, ANEF

The CNE® Test Plan lists the following for the area of Use Assessment and Evaluation Strategies:

Use Assessment and Evaluation Strategies

A. Provide input for the development of nursing program standards and policies regarding:
   1. admission
   2. progression
   3. graduation
B. Enforce nursing program standards related to
   1. admission
   2. progression
   3. graduation
C. Use a variety of strategies to assess and evaluate learning in these domains:
   1. cognitive
   2. psychomotor
   3. affective
D. Incorporate current research in assessment and evaluation practices.
E. Analyze available resources for learner assessment and evaluation.
F. Create assessment instruments to evaluate outcomes.
G. Use assessment instruments to evaluate outcomes.
H. Implement evaluation strategies that are appropriate to the learner and learning outcomes.
I. Analyze assessment and evaluation data.
J. Use assessment and evaluation data to enhance the teaching-learning process.
K. Advise learners regarding assessment and evaluation criteria.
L. Provide timely, constructive, and thoughtful feedback to learners.

The NLN CNE test plan Category 3 focuses on assessment and evaluation. As identified in *The Scope of Practice for Academic Nurse Educators* (NLN, 2012c), nurse educators use a multitude of strategies to assess and evaluate student learning. To maximize the effectiveness of these strategies, nurse educators:

- use extant literature to develop evidence-based assessment and evaluation practices
- use a variety of strategies to assess and evaluate learning in the cognitive, psychomotor, and affective domains
- implement evidence-based assessment and evaluation strategies that are appropriate to the learner and to learning goals

- use assessment and evaluation data to enhance the teaching-learning process
- provide timely, constructive, and thoughtful feedback to learners
- demonstrate skill in the design and use of tools for assessing clinical practice (NLN, 2012c, p. 17)

USE ASSESSMENT AND EVALUATION DATA TO ENHANCE THE TEACHING-LEARNING PROCESS; INCORPORATE CURRENT RESEARCH IN ASSESSMENT AND EVALUATION PRACTICES

Nurse educators are accountable for using evidence-based assessment and evaluation methods in classroom and clinical settings to maintain the quality of educational programs. Incorporating current research in assessment and evaluation practices provides a strong foundation for enhancing the teaching-learning process. Research evidence in empirical literature, white papers, position statements, and education-related references can help faculty to develop relevant assessment and evaluation strategies. For example, the *NLN Fair Testing Guidelines for Nursing Education* provides guidelines for use of standardized testing in assessment (NLN, 2012a). Reading current publications on developing assessment methods is essential for developing valid and reliable examinations and other assessment methods.

Teachers select appropriate strategies to assess achievement of learning in the cognitive, psychomotor, and affective domains while also using assessment and evaluation data to inform decisions about courses, programs, and curricula. These data are also used in determining educational standards, such as admission, progression, and graduation policies (Oermann & Gaberson, 2017).

Given the central nature of assessment and evaluation to nursing education, we must begin our discussion with a clarification of the definitions of these two terms. *Assessment* refers to measures that provide information about student abilities before, during, and after participation in programs (Billings & Halstead, 2016). Assessment includes both qualitative and quantitative data, which are used to provide feedback to students about their performance, as well as information and data for the educator to use in determining whether students have met student learning outcomes and competencies. Educators rely on assessment data to improve educational practices, strengthen programs, and develop educational policies.

The process of assessment is ongoing throughout the teaching/learning cycle. Assessment is used prior to developing programs, outcomes, and instructional methods. Preadmission testing is one means of assessment used to determine levels of students' needs and helps inform the ongoing development of the program and courses. Teachers modify instruction based on feedback attained through assessment of student learning. Figure 3.1 depicts this continuous and circular process.

Sometimes the word *measurement* is used interchangeably with the word *assessment*; it is not, however, synonymous. *Measurement* is a process of assigning numbers to represent student performance or achievement (Oermann & Gaberson, 2017). For example, a test score is a means for measuring the degree of student learning. Key to understanding this concept is recognizing that the ability to interpret measurement scores requires a frame of reference. Comparing one student's score or performance with others in a group, or *norm-referencing*, answers the question "how well does that student compare to others?" While grading on a curve is a much-used form of norm-referencing and can provide worthwhile assessment data, a disadvantage of this method is that it does not provide a means to judge student achievement in relationship to outcomes.

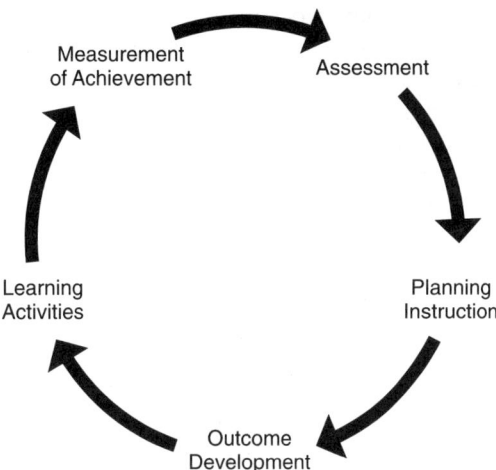

FIGURE 3.1 Interaction of assessment in planning, outcome development, learning strategies, and measuring achievement.

In contrast, *criterion-referencing* interprets scores based on preset criteria rather than on comparison to other students. This is sometimes referred to as *competency-based measurement*, in which achievement of a defined set of competencies measures student learning. For example, exam scores represent a criterion-referenced interpretation of student performance. Evaluation of performance of psychomotor skills often uses a criterion-referenced tool, such as a checklist or rubric to grade specific behaviors associated with the skill.

The second concept central to this discussion is *evaluation*. While a myriad of definitions address *evaluation*, in a basic sense, evaluating something means appraising its quality. Educational evaluation usually refers to a systematic appraisal of the quality of education. Because educators are accountable for evaluating the quality of the education they deliver, they are expected to use formal processes to perform a systematic evaluation of numerous areas, including student achievement of outcomes. To do so, educators use two major types of evaluation—*formative* and *summative*—and both are used in nursing programs. *Formative evaluation* occurs throughout the process of instruction, offering feedback about student progress with a goal of improving learning and clinical competency (Oermann & Gaberson, 2017). Formative evaluation allows teachers to continually assess student learning, which enables them to provide specific feedback about student performance and improve teaching strategies, the course, or the curriculum. During clinical instruction, teachers engage in ongoing observations used to guide the students' performance. Teachers may make immediate changes in instruction based on formative evaluation feedback, allowing students to modify their performance to achieve student learning outcomes.

Scenario 3.1

A clinical instructor observes that students are not following handwashing protocols on their first clinical day. The instructor decides to take 10 minutes at the end of the day to provide a brief handwashing refresher.

Consider: How might the instructor glean feedback from colleagues about similar performances in other clinical groups?

Summative evaluation occurs at the end of instruction and determines the overall achievement of the students in the course or at the end of the program. In essence, summative evaluation *sums up* or *summarizes* the outcome of the education. The final grade in a course is an example of summative evaluation; other examples of methods used for summative evaluation include exams, capstone projects, written assignments, portfolios, and practicum exams.

Program evaluation is an essential component of assuring quality in education. Teachers conduct assessment and evaluation activities continuously to improve learning, student outcomes, and program quality. Schools generally develop a lengthy systematic plan for evaluation that designates *what* will be evaluated, what assessment measures are used, *who* is responsible for completing the evaluation or gathering the data, *when* components are evaluated, and *how* results are reported. Regulatory agencies—such as the state board of nursing or state higher education boards and nursing discipline accrediting bodies—examine the school's evaluation plan to determine whether all aspects of the educational experience are evaluated and whether results are being used for ongoing curriculum and program improvement. The nurse educator is integral in the evaluation process and knowledgeable of the many elements of the school's evaluation plan.

PROVIDE INPUT FOR THE DEVELOPMENT OF NURSING PROGRAM STANDARDS AND POLICIES; ENFORCE NURSING PROGRAM STANDARDS

Educators are often called upon by their school's administration to provide input into student policies for admission, progression, and graduation. Basing these policies and decisions on relevant evidence supports high-quality education and student outcomes.

Admission Policies

Admission policies typically include a series of basic requirements, such as:

1. graduation from an approved or accredited program that provides the basic foundation for the program, that is, graduation from high school for a student seeking admission to a prelicensure nursing program;
2. a minimum required GPA in previous education;
3. a minimum score on a standardized entry examination;
4. ability to read and write English if it is not the native language of the applicant;
5. submission of official transcripts; and
6. relevant prerequisites, such as an RN license for registered nurse applicants seeking admission to an RN-BSN or graduate nursing program.

Some requirements, such as verification of completion of programs by providing official transcripts and proof of RN licensure, may be mandated by regulatory agencies such as boards of nursing, accrediting bodies, and higher education boards.

The nurse educator may be part of a committee that determines admission policies and/or approves applicants for admission. The purpose of these policies is to create meaningful criteria that facilitate the selection and approval processes, ultimately enabling admissions officials to determine which applicants are the most qualified and most likely to graduate. Standardized tests—such as the ACT, SAT, or GRE, or nursing-specific entrance exams—may play a role in determining an applicant's eligibility for admission as schools attempt to predict ultimate success.

> ### Scenario 3.2
>
> Faculty on the admissions committee are charged with developing preadmission testing criteria for their prelicensure RN program. They have contacted several companies that produce preadmission testing materials and have asked colleagues from other schools about their preadmission testing policies.
>
> *Consider:* What other resources might they consider when making their selection?

Progression Policies

Schools have policies that regulate progression within a program. For example, a policy may state that a student must achieve a minimum grade of C in a nursing course to progress to the next nursing course or to graduation. The minimum grade earned in nursing courses required for progression is often higher than for nonnursing courses. Additional data used to determine progression for prelicensure nursing programs might include satisfactory performance in clinical, grades on a dosage calculation examination, and successful performance of psychomotor skills. Graduate nursing programs may focus on other types of assessment measures to establish progression, such as successful completion of a predetermined number of clinical hours, documentation of accurate patient decisions related to advanced practice, and research activities.

Policies might regulate how many times a student may fail or withdraw from a course before being dismissed from the program. Some programs require students to complete all graduation requirements within a specific time period. Programs may use standardized tests to determine student progression between courses and levels. The practice of using standardized testing to determine a student's progression is controversial. Some state boards of nursing place restrictions on this practice.

All decisions related to progression (and other nursing policies) should be based on data. Consider Scenario 3.3, which depicts evaluation with the goal of informing a decision on a progression policy.

Graduation Policies

Graduation policies usually include stipulations that a student has successfully met program student learning outcomes, has completed all course work with a minimum GPA, and has met all financial obligations to the school.

Graduation policies may also include high-stakes testing, requiring students to attain a certain score on a standardized examination to graduate from a program.

> ### Scenario 3.3
>
> The faculty members at your school are examining data related to student success on the NCLEX. Specific percentages earned for each of the nursing courses were tracked and then correlated with the students' success on the NCLEX. Faculty determined that 10 students out of 100 graduating with the cohort failed the NCLEX. The students who failed the NCLEX scored an average of 78 percent in each of the nursing courses. Faculty used this information to reset the passing percentage for nursing courses from 75 percent to 80 percent.
>
> *Consider:* What additional actions might the faculty consider?

> **BOX 3.1 Excerpts from the NLN Fair Testing Guidelines for Nursing Education**
>
> Certainly, standardized test results are useful in various ways. They provide students with information about their knowledge compared to other students, using national norms; and they help faculty identify curricular strengths and weaknesses. But requiring a predetermined score for students to graduate and/or take the NCLEX in order to ensure that program pass rates remain at state board-prescribed levels is especially problematic for those who have successfully passed all other components of the nursing program. Students who cannot achieve the predetermined score may be forced to take the exit examination repeatedly until they achieve the score. They may fail the nursing course in which the test is a required component and endanger their standing in the nursing program. They may be denied their degrees or authorization to take the NCLEX. Cases like these can adversely affect the students and their families economically, i.e., while licensing is postponed, full salary potential is in jeopardy.
>
> **The Guidelines in Brief**
> 1. Faculty have an ethical obligation to ensure that both tests and the decisions based on tests are valid, supported by solid evidence, consistent across courses, and fair to all test takers regardless of age, gender, disability, race, ethnicity, national origin, religion, sexual orientation, linguistic background, testing style and ability, or other personal characteristics.
> 2. Faculty have the responsibility to assess students' abilities and assure that they are competent to practice nursing, while recognizing that current approaches to learning assessment are limited and imperfect.
> 3. Multiple sources of evidence are needed to evaluate basic nursing competence. Multiple approaches for assessment of knowledge and clinical abilities are particularly critical when high stakes decisions (such as progression or graduation) are based on the assessment.
> 4. Tests and other evaluative measures should be used not only to evaluate student achievement, but, as importantly, to support student learning, improve teaching, and guide program improvements.
> 5. Comprehensive testing, administration, and evaluation information must be readily available to faculty before they administer, grade, and distribute results from, or write policies related to, the use of standardized tests. Faculty have the responsibility to review and incorporate these materials in communications to students about standardized testing and its consequences.

Many schools have implemented high-stakes testing as part of their progression and graduation policies in an attempt to predict success on the NCLEX-RN®. However, this practice is not without concern. The National League for Nursing (NLN) assembled a group of nursing and evaluation experts to study this practice. In February, 2012, the NLN Board of Governors issued a document titled *The Fair Testing Imperative in Nursing Education* (NLN, 2012b). Box 3.1 contains excerpts from this document. It is important for faculty to read the entire document prior to making decisions about using standardized examinations in their programs.

USE A VARIETY OF STRATEGIES TO ASSESS AND EVALUATE LEARNING ACROSS DOMAINS

Assessment and evaluation of learner achievement is designed to determine whether students have met intended objectives and learning outcomes, and whether they have acquired the knowledge, skills, and abilities identified in the

Table 3.1

Bloom's Taxonomy and Domains of Learning

Domain	Level (Highest to Lowest)
Cognitive	Creating Evaluating Analyzing Applying Understanding Remembering
Psychomotor	Naturalization Articulation Precision Manipulation Imitation
Affective	Internalizing the values Understanding the concept Conceptualizing and organizing Valuing Responding Receiving

course, program, and curriculum (Billings & Halstead, 2016). When selecting assessment and evaluation methods, the teacher chooses methods that best reflect the intended learning outcome. This ensures that the assessment and evaluation strategies are valid because they are measuring what they are intended to measure.

Considerations when selecting assessment strategies include determining the setting for instruction and assessment, that is, classroom or clinical site, as well as the domain of learning assessed. Bloom's classic taxonomy (1956), updated in 2001 by Anderson and Krathwohl, depicts the level of behavior at which competencies are demonstrated. Bloom addressed the domains of learning, including the cognitive, psychomotor, and affective domains. In the cognitive domain, the emphasis is on acquisition and use of knowledge, with levels ranging in a hierarchy from least to most complex, that is, from remembering to creating (Table 3.1). In the psychomotor domain, the focus is on performance of manual or physical skills ranging from imitation to naturalization at the highest level. The affective domain incorporates emotions or feelings; the concept ranges from receiving to internalizing values.

Teachers assessing learning in the cognitive domain commonly use objective tests and written assignments. The psychomotor domain provides a foundation for skills attainment in nursing. It is most often assessed in the college skills laboratory, simulation laboratory, and clinical application in a health care setting.

The affective domain, while sometimes more difficult to assess than the other two domains, is important in nursing education. Students often demonstrate learning in the affective domain through the use of creative writing, portfolios, and reflective journals.

Clinical settings provide a venue where multiple domains may be assessed within a single experience. For example, a student caring for a patient who has an acute exacerbation of a severe illness may use critical thinking and decision-making

---

Scenario 3.4

Faculty in a nursing fundamentals course are discussing how to assess student under-standing of handwashing skills. They decide to develop a short quiz to test their cognitive understanding and plan to have the students demonstrate handwashing techniques in the skills lab to assess their psychomotor skills.

Consider: Is there a means for testing the affective domain on this topic?

---

skills to determine treatment (cognitive), perform a procedure (psychomotor), and demonstrate professionalism and empathy when working with the patient and the patient's family (affective).

CREATE ASSESSMENT INSTRUMENTS TO EVALUATE OUTCOMES

Teachers are responsible for developing assessment and evaluation strategies that yield meaningful data about student achievement and the effectiveness of the program. Assessment methods are designed to align with the lesson objectives and course student learning outcomes (both content and level of thinking). For example, an objective in a beginning clinical nursing course laboratory assignment states, "The learner will accurately measure a patient's vital signs." An appropriate measure of performance is to have the student demonstrate assessment of vital signs on a partner or simulation manikin.

Methods must be valid and measure what students should have learned in the course. For example, if novice students are learning about the nursing process, a valid assessment method might include asking the students to describe the steps in the nursing process. Assessment strategies must also be reliable, or consistent, and produce similar results whenever the instrument is used. For example, all clinical sections of a course use the same measurement tools so that all students are evaluated using the same criteria no matter who the clinical faculty might be. A consistent application of measurement in this instance supports interrater reliability.

USE ASSESSMENT INSTRUMENTS TO EVALUATE OUTCOMES; IMPLEMENT EVALUATION STRATEGIES APPROPRIATE TO THE LEARNER AND LEARNING OUTCOMES; ANALYZE AVAILABLE RESOURCES FOR LEARNER ASSESSMENT AND EVALUATION CRITERIA

Numerous instruments are available to evaluate learner attainment of outcomes. Whether assessing clinical or classroom performance, faculty should critically analyze available resources used in learner assessment and evaluation. Methods and instruments should meet the following guidelines:

1. Measurement methods must be valid and reliable.
2. Assessment methods should measure achievement of learning competencies or outcomes.
3. Learning objectives and outcomes must be measurable.

Various assessment measures are used to determine attainment of outcomes. Multiple types of evaluation methods result in increased information

Table 3.2

Sample Grading Rubric for Nursing Diagnosis and Nursing
Actions Assignment

Criteria	Criteria Unmet 0 Points	Criteria Partially Met 1 Point	Criteria Met 2 Points
Correctly states 1 nursing diagnosis	Nursing diagnosis was not present	Nursing diagnosis was present but not correctly stated	Nursing diagnosis was present and correctly stated
Correctly states 3 nursing actions	Less than 3 nursing actions identified	Three nursing actions present, but not correctly stated	Three nursing actions were present and correctly stated

and feedback, especially in formative evaluation, where it is possible to modify instruction as a result of assessment data.

Grading Rubrics

Grading rubrics assess student performance of subjective assignments using specific, measurable criteria. Typically, a grading rubric contains criteria that guide the student regarding the level of expectations for the assignment and guide the teacher in grading the assignment. These criteria include a description of each area evaluated, the level of performance for each grading point, and an associated score. The most essential characteristics of a robust and meaningful rubric are that the data collected are measurable and directly connected to the student learning outcomes that the assignment is designed to measure. Table 3.2 presents a sample rubric for a simple nursing diagnosis and plan of action assignment with a grading rubric.

Assessing Clinical Performance, Psychomotor Skills, and Affective Behaviors

Assessing clinical performance, psychomotor skills, and affective behaviors requires different methods of measurement than evaluating classroom performance. Clinical evaluation is complex and affected by numerous factors, many outside of the control of the faculty. Patient acuity, staffing levels, rapidly changing patient conditions, number and level of students, and clinical learning outcomes all impact straightforward evaluation of student performance in the clinical area. Subsequently, teachers use formative evaluation during the clinical course to provide ongoing feedback throughout the clinical day and adjust to student learning needs.

Clinical evaluation instruments are developed to provide specific, measurable criteria consistent with course student learning outcomes (Bonnel, 2016). According to Bonnel, primary strategies for evaluating clinical practice include observation, oral communication, written communication, simulation, and self-evaluation. Observation allows the teacher to witness student performance and may complement the use of checklists and anecdotal notes to support assessment data collected. Grading rubrics are commonly used to evaluate clinical performance, depicting a range from satisfactory to unsatisfactory, or points on a numerical scale to rate student achievement.

In the era of high-fidelity clinical simulators, scenarios and case studies have become a universal method for both practice and evaluation. Measurement of

---

Scenario 3.5

An experienced teacher is coaching a novice clinical faculty member who had asked for advice about a nursing student's performance. The student is not meeting clinical objectives and is in danger of failing the clinical experience. The student has been late for clinical, has not completed a plan of care, and could not state the side-effects of medications the student was to administer.

Consider: What advice would you give the novice educator about how to best assess the performance of this student?

---

cognitive, affective, and psychomotor behaviors ranging from simple to complex may be accomplished with the use of clinical simulation. Case studies and patient scenarios can provide realistic environments for care, enhanced by multimedia equipment that yields immediate feedback, allows for unlimited practice in a safe environment, and enables self-evaluation.

Assessing affective behaviors may be challenging, but a number of methods have been used effectively in nursing education for this purpose. Student self-assessment is a method used in a variety of educational settings, including the classroom, clinical, and nursing laboratories. Reflection on a learning experience is an affective behavior that allows students to consider their own performance based on assignment learning outcomes. Reflective journals and portfolios support self-assessment and may be used to demonstrate higher-level and abstract thinking. Clinical portfolios are used as a means to collect a collage of artifacts that reflect learning and achievement over time.

Classroom Assessment

Classroom assessment is accomplished through a variety of strategies to assess student achievement of learning outcomes. Assignments such as papers, debates, audio and video recordings, presentations, group projects, journals, simulation and gaming, portfolios, reflection, role-play, service learning, and concept mapping are all used to assess and evaluate student learning.

Developing Valid and Reliable Tests

In *The Scope of Practice for Academic Nurse Educators* (2012c), the NLN states that teaching, learning, and evaluation strategies are evidence based. Creating valid and reliable tests, and using standard metrics to examine outcomes of testing, provide the nurse educator with evidence of dependable measures that yield a high level of confidence in the results. Faculty must have confidence that the evaluation methods yield an accurate measure of the students' achievement of the learning outcomes. An important task of faculty is to eliminate irrelevant variance from these measures. That is, the results obtained from the instruments used to evaluate student learning are not influenced by any factors other than the students' learning. Eliminating all irrelevant variance is impossible but should be the goal when developing and using evaluation instruments.

Constructing valid and reliable tests requires skill, practice, and time. When planning to test students, the teacher first determines the purpose of the testing. If the test is administered prior to instruction, it may reflect readiness or placement. When administered during instruction, it serves as a formative evaluation of learning. When administered at the conclusion of instruction, the test serves as summative evaluation of learning, and may supply information to determine progression and grading (Billings, 2016). Numerous tools assist the teacher in test development, including test blueprints, test storage and retrieval databases, and test analysis software.

Test Blueprints

Development of a test blueprint, a map that connects content and outcomes to the test items, is one method used to address content validity of an exam. Faculty develop a test blueprint prior to creating an exam and include the course/unit outcome, the content, expected cognitive level (Bloom's taxonomy), total number of desired test items, and weight or percentage of the exam allotted to each area. An additional consideration is the level of difficulty of items, which should correlate with the cognitive level of the learning outcome. When testing prelicensure nursing students, categories may be added that reflect the NCLEX-RN test plan and components of the nursing process.

Numerous examples of tables and spreadsheets, including some that are computer generated, are available for nurse educators to use when developing a test blueprint. Table 3.3 depicts a sample test blueprint, relating content areas to the nursing process, assigning weight to each area, and classifying according to cognitive level. This blueprint is a summative type of test blueprint. Another type of blueprint tracks each test item to specifics important to the teacher. Table 3.4 provides an example of a test blueprint that demonstrates congruency among the test item, lesson objective, and course student learning outcomes. This type of test blueprint is preferred because it demonstrates a higher level of specificity for the validity of the test items.

When selecting the number of test items, the teacher takes into account a number of considerations, including the level of the student and the time available for testing. While test reliability may increase with the number of test items, there may be time limitations. A general guideline is to allow approximately one minute per multiple-choice test item. Items that require higher-level thinking may need more time to answer than those that test a lower level of thinking.

Table 3.3

Sample Test Blueprint Using Nursing Process Content Areas on a 100-Item Exam

Outcome/ Content Area	Percentage of Exam in Content Area	Cognitive Level: Knowledge	Cognitive Level: Comprehension	Cognitive Level: Application
Assessment	25%	8	8	9
Diagnosis	20%	6	6	8
Planning	15%	4	4	7
Intervention	15%	4	4	7
Evaluation	25%	8	8	9
Total	100%	30	30	40

Table 3.4

Test Blueprint Aligning Test Items to the Lesson Objective and Course Student Learning Outcome

Question	Lesson Objective	Course Student Learning Outcome	Step in the Nursing Process	Other Nursing Situation	Detailed Objective on the NCLEX® Test Plan	Cognitive Level	Difficulty Level of Key	Item Discrimination of Key
1								
2								
3								
4								
5								
6								
7								
8								
9								
10								
11								
Etc.								

Copyright 2016 Linda Caputi, Inc. Used with permission from www.LindaCaputi.com

Test Construction and Item Writing

Objective tests assess understanding of content and the ability to think at the remembering, understanding, applying, and analyzing levels. Test items are designed to measure competency or mastery of a subject. Objective-style examinations permit testing a number of students at one time and may be scored rapidly, often with the use of computerized scoring equipment that offers item analysis. Disadvantages of objective testing include the difficulty in writing items that examine critical thinking skills as well as the time needed to develop valid, reliable tests.

Developing and selecting the format for test items is time-consuming, requiring skill and practice. However, writing good, reliable test items is part of the faculty's role responsibilities. Item format is determined by considering which of the multiple types of formats most directly measures the intended learning outcome (Billings, 2016). The most common item formats are multiple-choice, true-false, matching, short-answer, fill-in-the-blank, and ordered-response. Another form of multiple-choice, labeled *multiple-response*, includes several correct responses. The NCLEX-RN uses alternative-format questions, including fill-in-the-blank, multiple-response, drag-and-drop, ordered-response, picture/graphic, and audio questions. The National Council of State Boards of Nursing (NCSBN) is currently working on developing new item types. The Next-Generation NCLEX (NGN) will include these new items that are directly focused on measuring clinical judgment. This is an area of testing that all faculty need to monitor. This change in item types is to better measure whether the candidate can engage in thinking in the same way that nurses are required to think in actual practice. This new examination promises to be much more challenging than the current format. Faculty must learn how to teach clinical judgment first, then apply clinical judgment to nursing practice, and, finally, to write items that reflect the proposed item types (Caputi, 2018, 2019; Dickison et al., 2016).

Regardless of the format selected, exams should include high-level, critical-thinking test items. According to McDonald (2018), test items should require students to draw on their nursing knowledge, analyze the problem from multiple viewpoints, and apply concepts that propose the most appropriate solution to the problem. Critical-thinking tests should be at the application or higher cognitive level, and require higher-level thinking skills to determine the correct answers.

Multiple-choice test items typically are composed of the question, referred to as the *stem*, and a set of responses, with the correct response referred to as the *key* and the incorrect responses as *distracters*. When writing the stem, the teacher should use clear, unbiased language and avoid giving overt clues to the correct answer. Each response should be plausible and approximately the same length and level of complexity. All items should be referenced in the test blueprint and should be checked for accuracy.

ANALYZE ASSESSMENT AND EVALUATION DATA

Collecting data is the first step of the assessment and evaluation process; subsequent careful analysis of the data is critical to performing evidence-based assessment. Teachers use multiple means of measuring student performance, then accurately interpret the data to produce an indicator of student learning that is reliable. Understanding test results may be challenging and requires knowledge of some basic concepts as well as experience to gain skill and confidence in interpreting results.

Analyzing Test Results

One of the most important aspects of testing is completion of a statistical analysis. The purpose of completing a statistical analysis on test items is to ensure that exams effectively evaluate student learning. Important measures of exam analysis include the difficulty level of test items, item discrimination for all answers, and the reliability of the overall exam.

Many nursing programs rely on the use of test scoring software to assist with test development, storage, blueprinting, and analysis. With the ease of using these systems, the manual calculation of test item statistics is eliminated. It is, however, extremely important for teachers to understand the reports generated by the testing software.

Difficulty Level

When evaluating exam results, the teacher first considers whether the examination was too difficult or too easy. Exam difficulty may be determined through reviewing the mean, median, and mode. The mean is the average of the group scores on the exam, the median is the halfway point at which one-half of the students scored above this number and one-half scored below, and the mode is the most frequently obtained score.

To effectively measure different levels of student learning, exams include items of varying levels of difficulty. Item difficulty (p value), also called the *difficulty level*, *difficulty factor*, or *difficulty index*, measures the percent of students that answered a test item correctly. The range would be reported as 0.00 to 1.00. For example, a difficulty factor of 0.79 means that 79 percent of the students answered an item correctly. According to McDonald (2018), an acceptable range for an item's p value would be .70 to .80, although both easier (p value above .80) and more difficult (p value below .70) questions may be included in an exam. The mean p value (p value of all items on a test) indicates the average percent correct on the test.

Item Discrimination

The second area to consider when evaluating test results is to determine whether the item discriminated between those students who knew the content and those who did not. Those who knew the content and those who did not is determined by the grade earned on that exam. For each item, this statistic reflects how those students who scored highest on the exam answered that item. The item discrimination factor compares the number of students who answered the item correctly based on their overall score on the exam to those who did not score as well.

An effective exam question will discriminate between the students who have scored at a higher level and those individuals scoring at a lower level. For example, if students with high test scores answer an item correctly and students with low overall test scores answer the item incorrectly, the item is said to *discriminate*, or *differentiate*, between those who do and those who do not know the material. If, however, a larger number of low-scoring students on the exam answered the question correctly than high-scoring students, the question is not reliable in differentiating between those who know and those who do not know the material.

Two methods for item discrimination include the item discrimination index (DI—sometimes called the *discrimination index*), and the point biserial index (PBI), sometimes referred to as the *point biserial correlation coefficient* (McDonald, 2018). Although the DI is more easily calculated, the PBI is the more commonly used measurement of item discrimination, as it is produced by most test analysis software.

The DI assesses high-scoring and low-scoring student responses to test items. An acceptable level for the DI is 25 percent. The DI is calculated by considering the top percent and bottom percent of the student scores as follows:

$$DI = a - b$$

a = response frequency (percent) of the top scoring students on an item
b = response frequency (percent) of the lowest scoring students on an item

For example, if 75 percent of the top-scoring students answered an item correctly, and 50 percent of the lowest-scoring students answered an item correctly, the DI is 25 percent, that is, DI = 75 percent − 50 percent = 25 percent.

The most accurate measure of an item's level of discrimination is its PBI. Test analysis software is available to assist the teacher in quickly determining the PBI; thus, calculating this manually is rare. Instead, it is more important to be able to interpret analysis reports correctly than spending time with manual calculations.

The PBI ranges from −1.00 to 1.00, where a positive (+) point biserial for the correct answer (the key) indicates that high-scoring students answered a test

Table 3.5

Interpreting Individual Item Results

Individual Item Statistics					
Item Number	**Difficulty (*p* value)**	**Overall Item PBI**	**Option**[a]	**% of Students Choosing Each Response Option**	**PBI**
1	0.70	0.42	A	0.03	−0.46
			B	0.22	−0.30
			C	0.70	0.42
			D	0.05	−0.28
2	0.75	0.09	**A**	0.75	0.09
			B	0.08	−0.28
			C	0.11	0.08
			D	0.06	−0.26

[a]The correct answer or the key is in bold.

item correctly more frequently than low-scoring students and a negative (−) point biserial for the key indicates that low-scoring students answered a test item correctly more frequently than high-scoring students. The higher the PBI, the better the item discriminates between low and high achievers on an examination (McDonald, 2018). McDonald states that a PBI above 0.20 defines a highly discriminating item on an exam, adding that items with a PBI of lower than 0.20 should be revised. A zero PBI indicates that students who did well and those who did poorly on the exam answered the item correctly with equal frequency. Items that are very easy or very difficult will have a low discrimination level. All wrong answers, or the distracters, should have a negative PBI, which indicates that more low-scoring students selected the distracter than high-scoring students.

In addition to analyzing overall PBI for each test item, the teacher also critically examines each item's details, that is, the difficulty (*p* value) and PBI of the distracters for each test item. See Table 3.5 for examples of results of two test items.

Item 1 in Table 3.5 represents a statistically stable question: the item difficulty of 0.70 and the PBI of 0.42 reflect that the item discriminated well between high-scoring and low-scoring students. The negative PBI on each of the incorrect items indicates that low-scoring students selected the incorrect items more frequently than the high-scoring students. A different picture is reflected in item 2. While the difficulty level of 0.75 is sufficient, the correct response is shown to be a poor discriminator, with a PBI of 0.09, with distracter C also having a positive PBI. The teacher would consider accepting answer C in this case and should modify the item before using it again. For both items, all distracters were selected by students taking the exam. This is a positive finding. If there are distracters that no students chose, then the distracter is not distracting the uninformed student and is not functioning as a distracter. If there are four options and no students choose one of the options because it is obviously wrong, students now have a one in three chance of correctly guessing the answer rather than a one in four chance. This makes the item less reliable if the chance for guessing the correct answer is increased. Therefore, distracters that are not selected by any students should be rewritten or eliminated. These distracters are causing the student to spend time reading them but are not functioning for the purpose for which they were intended.

Scenario 3.6

The faculty are examining results of a recent multiple-choice test. They are pleased to see that the mean *p* value was .94, and most of the students were happy as well. However, as they looked at the item analysis, they saw that many items had a low PBI, and even the low-scoring students did not select the distracters.

Consider:
1. Is there a problem with the faculty being pleased with a *p* value of .94?
2. What might the faculty consider before using this test in the future?

Reliability

Finally, when examining test results, the teacher asks, "What is the reliability of the exam?" Reliability refers to the consistency of test results (McDonald, 2018). There are a number of measures of reliability, including test-retest, parallel-form, and internal consistency.

Test-retest reliability requires administering the identical test to the same individual on a second occasion and then determining the correlation between the scores. In parallel-form reliability, two different forms of the test are administered to the same person, with the results of the two tests then being correlated. Both of these methods are unfeasible for most classroom teachers owing to time constraints and difficulty in creating equivalent forms of a test.

When considering internal consistency and reliability, the Kuder-Richardson Formula 20 (KR-20) may be used to measure interitem consistency. As with the PBI, the range of the KR-20 will fall between –1.0 and 1.0, where a reliability coefficient of 1.0 indicates perfect reliability and a reliability coefficient of 0.0 indicates that the test lacks reliability. It would be rare to see a negative KR-20, as this would mean that many of the test items are being answered correctly by low-scoring students instead of high-scoring students. A KR-20 score of 0.60 is acceptable for teacher-made nursing examinations.

Using Standardized Exams

Many schools of nursing use commercially available tests to supplement faculty-developed exams. Standardized tests have become a common means of demonstrating evaluation of programs and are frequently found on a nursing program's systematic evaluation plan. When selecting these exams, faculty carefully consider a number of variables, including detailed information about content and how the content to include on the examination was determined, data on validity and reliability, and the level of competence tested. It is important that faculty ask these important questions before using a standardized exam. Faculty often discuss the attributes of various commercial exams with other users and find that anecdotal information about exams, as well as the support offered by the test agency, will influence purchasing decisions. Another important question faculty should ask is why is standardized testing needed? Faculty's responsibility is to provide a solid curriculum, expert teaching, quality assessment and evaluation methods, and remediation to help students succeed based on the results of the evaluation methods used. If these are all in place, faculty should question why testing from an outside company is needed. Faculty due diligence requires answers to this question before mandating that students spend time and money on an additional product that may not be needed. Finally, if it is determined that standardized testing is needed, faculty should address the problems with in-house testing and attempt to fix the problems first. Once the attempt is made, faculty should then determine whether standardized testing is still needed. The *NLN Fair Testing Guidelines* suggest that faculty seek out and learn the practices of schools who do not implement high-stakes standardized testing in their programs. Perhaps changes to the program's curriculum, teaching, assessment and evaluation methods, and remediation can correct deficiencies so that purchase of an outside examination may not be required. Faculty must consider the burden of time and expense of standardized testing for the student; therefore, good rationale and evidence for using standardized testing is imperative.

ADVISE LEARNERS REGARDING ASSESSMENT AND EVALUATION CRITERIA

Faculty members are responsible for apprising students of the criteria on which they will be evaluated. In some instances, this is communicated through academic bulletins or handbooks that outline formal policies related to course expectations, academic progression, standardized testing, and clinical expectations. Course syllabi should clearly define these expectations, providing clear descriptions and expectations of assignments and evaluation methods.

Distributing test blueprints, detailed assignment grading rubrics, and clearly delineated expectations to learners supports both the student and faculty conducting the assessment. If clinical evaluation is part of the course, students are provided objective, measurable performance criteria to guide their behavior.

Straightforward communication of all expectations to students supports positive outcomes and helps avoid confusion and misunderstanding. Transparency regarding assessment and evaluation criteria also supports the delivery of growth-producing feedback to students.

PROVIDE TIMELY, CONSTRUCTIVE, AND THOUGHTFUL FEEDBACK TO LEARNERS

Formative evaluation, as previously mentioned, is used to supply feedback to support learning. When providing student feedback, the teacher considers a number of criteria. Feedback should be timely, specific, and constructive. Effective feedback is given as close to the time of assessment as possible, allowing students to modify their behavior and respond to a learning experience. Feedback should contain specific information for the student to use to improve performance and should address both strengths and areas for development as well as what steps to take to achieve expected outcomes. Constructive feedback focuses on specific ways to improve performance.

In addition to written assignments and examinations, midterm and/or end-of-term conferences may be used to discuss performance and are a common practice in the clinical learning environment. The content discussed about clinical performance should be concrete and specific. It is important to focus on specific behaviors, including what is right, what is wrong, why it is wrong, and how the behavior may be corrected. For example, it would be better to tell a student, "In performing the patient's dressing change, you did not follow sterile technique. You contaminated the site with your sleeve, and your hair was in the sterile field," rather than, "You need to improve your sterile technique." When students perform poorly or demonstrate unsafe behaviors in the clinical area, the teacher should immediately meet with the student to discuss the performance and create a plan for improvement. For unsafe behaviors, close supervision is required until the faculty determines that the student is providing safe patient care.

SUMMARY

Assessment and evaluation data inform decisions about courses, programs, curricula, and educational standards and policies. Nurse educators are accountable for understanding and using evidence-based assessment and evaluation methods in all learning environments. A variety of evaluation strategies should be used in measuring all domains of learning. Many strategies support assessment and evaluation of learner outcomes across learning domains.

Practice Test Questions

1. NCLEX scores for the nursing program have been falling and the faculty are considering implementing a required exit test. Which statement best reflects faculty understanding of fair testing guidelines?
    A. "We need to consider all the data before developing an exit test policy."
    B. "NCLEX scores will go up if we require the students to retake the test to achieve the benchmark score."
    C. "Standardized tests have proven results and predict who will pass the NCLEX."
    D. "Students should be able to demonstrate a high score on the standardized test before we let them take the NCLEX."

2. A nurse faculty member on a clinical unit notices that the students are not correctly documenting their patient's vital signs. He develops a short exercise to be used in that day's post-conference to practice vital sign documentation. This is an example of which type of assessment?
    A. Criterion-referenced assessment
    B. Summative assessment
    C. Norm-referenced assessment
    D. Formative assessment

3. Which best represents the purpose of a summative clinical evaluation tool?
    A. Determination of the relative effect of education on the students' weekly clinical performance
    B. Assessment of students' acquisition of knowledge and skills during a particular clinical experience
    C. Determination that learning occurred and behavioral objectives were met during the semester
    D. Assessment of all activities associated with students' clinical experience over the duration of the program

4. Which best describes a criterion-referenced assessment activity?
    A. Interpretation of data in terms of a norm or group
    B. Evaluation of mastery of specified outcomes
    C. Use of information for predictive purposes
    D. Comparison of data between groups

5. The graduate nursing faculty are considering an evaluation method that demonstrates *summative* end-of-program student achievement of program learning outcomes. Which assessment method would be the best choice?
    A. Cumulative portfolio assignments in each course
    B. A comprehensive final course exam
    C. A reflective journal
    D. Self-evaluation reflection survey

6. Faculty in a nursing fundamentals course are developing assignments. To assess the objective "Understand the concepts of asepsis and sterile technique," which assignment is best?
   A. Demonstrate a sterile dressing change in the lab.
   B. Develop an essay on asepsis and sterile technique.
   C. Administer a short-answer quiz on asepsis and sterile technique.
   D. Create a poster showing how to change a sterile dressing.

7. The clinical faculty member wants to determine students' ability to perform sterile technique. To assess the objective "The student will be able to demonstrate the process of sterile technique in changing a dressing," which measurement is the best choice?
   A. Administer a short-answer quiz.
   B. Ask students to verbalize the steps of a sterile dressing change.
   C. Have students write 2 to 3 paragraphs about changing sterile dressings.
   D. Ask students to show how to change a sterile dressing.

8. The teacher decides to use a reflective journal as an assessment measure in a clinical course. This method is most effective in measuring which learning domain?
   A. Affective
   B. Cognitive
   C. Summative
   D. Psychomotor

9. The faculty member wants to assess the students' ability to apply the nursing process to a case study scenario and is developing test questions related to the case. Which question stem best assesses the ability to apply the nurse process?
   A. Describe the parts of the nursing process.
   B. Prioritize the actions of the nurse in this case.
   C. Which nursing diagnosis applies to this case?
   D. When should the nurse notify the physician?

10. To assess the students' ability to meet the objective "Define terms related to isolation precautions," which assignment is best?
    A. Group discussion
    B. Demonstration of isolation precautions
    C. Short essay
    D. Matching exercise

11. The nurse educator is writing a test question to assess the students' ability to apply theory to practice in the care of a patient with a neurological disorder. Which stem represents an application-level question?
    A. List the cranial nerves.
    B. Identify the steps in completing a neurological assessment.
    C. Prioritize the nursing actions for a patient having a seizure.
    D. State the precautions that are needed when caring for a patient with a seizure disorder.

12. The course faculty have developed a 100-item final exam. Which objective is most likely to be met by this type of assessment?
   A. Demonstrate comprehension of course concepts.
   B. Apply critical thinking in patient care settings.
   C. Demonstrate achievement of outcomes through self-reflection.
   D. Provide a comprehensive assessment of multiple patients.

13. A nursing course is taught by three faculty members who share responsibility for classroom content, laboratory time, and clinical experiences. When evaluating students in this course, what must the faculty do to ensure that students are receiving a fair grade?
   A. Hold weekly meetings of the faculty members to evaluate students.
   B. All students are evaluated by the same faculty member.
   C. Faculty members establish interrater reliability for the course evaluation strategies.
   D. Students are graded solely on a final exam prepared by all faculty in the course.

Exam Item	Difficulty Factor (*p* value)	Item Discrimination (Point Biserial Index)	Reliability (KR-20)
1	.72	0.39	0.80
2	.50	0.68	0.76

14. Considering the above item analysis, which statement is correct?
   A. The reliability of the items is poor.
   B. In item 2, the lower-scoring students answered the question correctly.
   C. The difficulty factor of both items is within an acceptable range.
   D. The item discrimination (PBI) indicates that the items discriminate well between low-scoring and high-scoring students.

Individual Item Statistics					
Item Number	Difficulty (*p* value)	Overall Item PBI	Option	Response Proportion	PBI of the key (correct answer)
1	.74	0.10	A	0.74	0.10
			B	0.08	−0.28
			C	0.12	0.08
			D	0.06	−0.26

15. Analyze the above item statistics. Based on this analysis, which statement is correct?
   A. Of the students, 74 percent answered the question correctly.
   B. More high-scoring students selected answer B than low-scoring students.
   C. More low-scoring students selected A than high-scoring students.
   D. This is a highly discriminating item.

Mean *p* Value	Kuder-Richardson (KR20)
.36	0.36

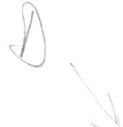

16. When interpreting the above statistics on an exam, what conclusion would you make?
   A. Test items discriminate well between high-scoring and low-scoring students.
   B. The test items' difficulty level and discrimination are correlated.
   C. Item difficulty and reliability are within acceptable ranges.
   D. The items are very difficult and the test lacks reliability.

17. The novice nurse educator is reviewing item analysis results from a recent examination. Which statement demonstrates that the educator understands the purpose of item analysis?
   A. "I want to find ways to give the students extra points."
   B. "I want to have proof so that the students can't argue with the results."
   C. "The results will show me how to make the test easier next time."
   D. "I am looking for items that may be too difficult, too easy, or had two correct answers."

18. A nursing instructor is reviewing the item analysis for an exam. For one item, the instructor sees the following analysis:

p Value	Answer	Response Proportion
1.00	A	0
	B	1.0
	C	0
	D	0

What is the best interpretation of the above results?
   A. The content was well covered in class.
   B. Only the higher-scoring students had the correct answer.
   C. No students selected the distractors.
   D. The item was too difficult and needs revision.

19. The teacher develops the following test question:
Respiratory precautions should be used for a client who has a disease transmitted by which of the following:
   a. Airborne droplet nuclei
   b. Bloodborne pathogens
   c. Poor handwashing technique
   d. Touching a contaminated object

Which Bloom's taxonomy level is being tested in the above item?
   A. Understanding
   B. Applying
   C. Analyzing
   D. Evaluating

20. The nursing instructor is preparing new items for an examination on neurological assessment for a health assessment course. Which stem measures learning at the analyzing level?

A. Which cranial nerve is being tested by observing the cardinal positions of gaze?

B. The nurse observes that the patient's tongue deviates to one side and there is right-sided hemiplegia. What other neurological tests can the nurse include in the assessment when assessing a patient with a CVA?

C. The nurse is initiating a care plan for a patient just admitted with Parkinson disease and aspiration pneumonia. Which of these nursing diagnoses should take priority?

D. Which of these statements by the mother of a child recently diagnosed with Duchenne dystrophy suggests the need for further teaching?

References

Anderson, L., & Krathwohl, D. (2001). *A taxonomy for learning, teaching, and assessing: A revision of Bloom's taxonomy of educational objectives*. New York: Longman.

Billings, D. (2016). Developing and using classroom tests. In D. M. Billings & J. A. Halstead (Eds.), *Teaching in nursing: A guide for faculty* (5th ed., pp. 423–426). St. Louis, MO: Elsevier.

Billings, D. M., & Halstead, J. A. (2016). *Teaching in nursing: A guide for faculty* (5th ed.). St. Louis, MO: Elsevier.

Bloom, B. S. (1956). *Taxonomy of educational objectives: The classification of educational goals*. New York: Longman.

Bonnel, W. (2016). Clinical performance evaluation. In D. M. Billings & J. A. Halstead (Eds.), *Teaching in nursing: A guide for faculty* (6th ed., pp. 443–462). St. Louis, MO: Elsevier.

Caputi, L. (2019). Guest Editorial. Reflections on the National Council of State Boards of Nursing's Next Generation NCLEX with implications for nursing programs. *Nursing Education Perspectives, 40*(1), 2–3.

Caputi, L. (2018). *Think like a nurse: A handbook*. Rolling Meadows, IL: Windy City Publisher.

Dickison, P., Luo, X., Kim, D., Woo, A., Muntean, W., & Bergstrom, B. (2016). Assessing higher-order cognitive constructs by using an information-process framework. *Journal of Applied Testing Technology, 17*(1), 1–19.

McDonald, M. E. (2018). *The nurse educator's guide to assessing learning outcomes* (4th ed.). Burlington, MA: Jones & Bartlett.

National League for Nursing (2012a). Fair testing guidelines for nursing education. Retrieved from http://www.nln.org/docs/default-source/default-document-library/fairtestingguidelines.pdf?sfvrsn=2

National League for Nursing (2012b). The fair testing imperative for nursing education. Retrieved from http://www.nln.org/docs/default-source/about/nln-vision-series-%28position-statements%29/nlnvision_4.pdf

National League for Nursing (2012c). *The scope of practice for academic nurse educators*. Philadelphia, PA: Lippincott Williams & Wilkins.

Oermann, M., & Gaberson, K. (2017). *Evaluation and testing in nursing education* (5th ed.). New York: Springer.

4

Participate in Curriculum Design and Evaluation of Program Outcomes

Linda Caputi, EdD, MSN, RN, CNE, ANEF

The CNE® Test Plan lists the following for the area of Participate in Curriculum Design and Evaluation of Program Outcomes:

Participate in Curriculum Design and Evaluation of Program Outcomes

A. Demonstrate knowledge of curriculum development, including:
    1. identifying program outcomes
    2. developing competency statements
    3. writing course objectives
    4. selecting appropriate learning activities
    5. selecting appropriate clinical experiences
    6. selecting appropriate evaluation strategies

B. Actively participate in the design of the curriculum to reflect:
    1. institutional philosophy and mission
    2. current nursing and health care trends
    3. community and societal needs
    4. nursing principles, standards, theory, and research
    5. educational principles, theory, and research
    6. use of technology

C. Lead the development of curriculum design.

D. Lead the development of course design.

E. Analyze results of program evaluation.

F. Revise the curriculum based on evaluation of:
    1. program outcomes
    2. learner needs
    3. societal and health care trends
    4. stakeholder feedback (e.g., from learners, agency personnel, accrediting agencies, advisory boards)

G. Implement curricular revisions using appropriate change theories and strategies.

H. Collaborate with community and clinical partners to support educational goals.

I. Design program assessment plans that promote continuous quality improvement.

J. Implement the program assessment plan.

K. Evaluate the program assessment plan.

The activities noted in the detailed CNE test blueprint reflect Competency 4 of the *Scope of Practice for Academic Nurse Educators* (National League for Nursing [NLN], 2012) related to the nurse educator's role in the important function of developing, implementing, and evaluating the nursing program curriculum. A primary role of the academic nurse educator is to participate in curriculum design and evaluation of program outcomes. The word *curriculum* may be defined in a number of ways. Faculty working together in a school of nursing should all use the same definition of the word *curriculum* as well as an understanding of what curriculum revision entails. This chapter covers the design, development, and evaluation of a curriculum and addresses the specific responsibilities of faculty as active participants in curriculum design and evaluation of program outcomes.

DEMONSTRATE KNOWLEDGE OF CURRICULUM DEVELOPMENT; ACTIVELY PARTICIPATE IN THE DESIGN OF THE CURRICULUM

Developing a curriculum is an organized, systematic process. The overall intent of a curriculum is to develop a program plan of study that results in graduates exhibiting characteristics reflective of what they learned in the nursing program. This requires determining the desired characteristics that students will display upon successful completion of all course work in the program. The nurse educator must have knowledge of the curriculum development/revision process and work from that basic understanding. Important to this work is intentionality (Emory, 2014). Faculty approach curriculum development in a thoughtful, intentional manner to create a program that educates safe, competent nurses. Intentionality also refers to making deliberate connections between student outcomes, the manner in which courses are structured, the content to be delivered, and how the curriculum will be taught. All tasks related to curriculum development are to ensure that students achieve the program student learning outcomes (SLOs).

The program SLOs are broad statements. Most nursing programs write from six to nine program SLOs. Because these SLOs are the intended outcomes of the program of study, they must be measured to ensure that they are achieved. Therefore, the beginning point is to write measurable SLOs as the end product of the program. However, because program SLOs are broad statements, they may be difficult to measure. Writing specific competencies for each program SLO provides detailed behaviors for each SLO; these competencies are measurable. The American Nurses Association (ANA) defines a competency as "an expected level of performance that integrates knowledge, skills, abilities, and judgment" (ANA, 2014). Table 4.1 presents an example program SLO with related competency statements. The specific competencies provide measurable behaviors to determine whether the

Table 4.1

Example Program Student Learning Outcome (SLO) with Related Competency Statements

Example Program SLO	Example Competencies for the SLO
Participate in quality improvement processes to improve patient care.	Apply quality improvement processes to effectively implement patient safety initiatives and monitor performance measures, including nursing-sensitive indicators.
	Analyze information gathered using quality improvement metrics to identify changes for improved patient outcomes.
	Identify gaps between local practice and best practice and provide recommendations for closing any gaps.
	Participate in analyzing errors and identifying system improvements.

student has met the program SLO of "Participate in quality improvement processes to improve patient care."

There are a number of sources that faculty can use to identify appropriate competencies as behaviors that align with program learning outcomes. Selected sources follow:

- National League for Nursing: *Outcomes and competencies for graduates of practical/ vocational, diploma, associate degree, baccalaureate, master's, practice doctorate, and research doctorate programs in nursing* (2010).
- American Association of College of Nursing: *The Essentials of Baccalaureate Education for Professional Nursing Practice* (2008), *The Essentials of Master's Education in Nursing* (2011), *The Essentials of Doctoral Education for Advanced Nursing Practice* (2006)
- Quality and Safety Education for Nurses competencies (QSEN.org, n.d.)
- Some states have developed nurse core competencies, such as the Maine Nurse Core Competencies (2013), available at https://www.omne.org/wp-content/uploads/2016/12/ME-RN-Competencies.pdf
- The detailed NCLEX-RN® and NCLEX-PN® test plans
- For graduate programs, competencies required for certification

Competencies published by professional organizations are a reliable source of information. However, these resources are not frequently updated. Therefore, it is important to review them for currency and check for any new updates.

An important source of competencies is from current practice. Nurse educators study the current health care environments that relate to the level of nurse they are educating and determine what current practice requires of new graduates. Practice changes frequently and rapidly. It is critical that all competencies reflect current practice. Further discussion of the basis for program SLOs follows.

THE BASIS FOR PROGRAM SLOs

If writing the program SLOs is the first step in development of a curriculum, the question is, "What is the basis for these program SLOs?" There are a number of important entities that faculty must consider when writing program SLOs (Caputi, 2010). Table 4.2 lists some of these important entities, accompanied by explanations.

Developing or revising curriculum requires a knowledge of professional standards—including nursing principles, standards of care, theory, and research—with implementation of each in the nursing program at the appropriate level for the type of nursing program. Faculty must make deliberate decisions about how these professional standards are used for the development of curriculum and how they are taught depending on the type of program: LPN, ADN, diploma, BSN, MSN, or DNP. The differentiated outcomes and competencies developed by the NLN (2010) are useful when making these decisions.

As indicated by this discussion, curriculum is no longer solely based on a nursing theorist or other established theoretical framework. Curriculum building is based on current nursing practice, the needs of the patients in the health care system, and a number of influencing initiatives. Although becoming outdated, some faculty may use the terms *organizing framework* or *theoretical framework* to represent the basis on which the curriculum is structured. Developing a curriculum that meets current health care needs requires faculty to maintain currency in both the practice and academic environments to ensure that the curriculum does

Table 4.2

Entities Faculty Must Consider When Writing Program Student Learning Outcomes (SLOs)

Important Entity	Explanation
The philosophy/mission/learning outcomes of the parent organization in which the nursing program resides	The institutional philosophy or mission that provides information about the focus of that institution and why it exists.
	May be expressed as value statements that provide overall direction for the philosophy/mission of the nursing program. General educational learning outcomes that all students graduating from that institution will achieve.
	The nursing program SLOs ensure that those general educational learning outcomes are met as an expression of the nursing program SLOs. For example, if an institution-level educational outcome is "Engage in critical thinking," a nursing program SLO might be "Engage in clinical judgment to provide quality patient care."
Regulatory requirements	State boards of nursing or other governmental agencies that develop requirements for the nursing program.
	There is a wide range of requirements among states.
	Some states provide very detailed curriculum requirements; others are not as detailed in their expectations related to curriculum, providing general guidelines to which nursing schools must comply.
Accreditation agencies	Nursing accreditation agencies include the Commission for Nursing Education Accreditation (CNEA), the Accreditation Commission for Education in Nursing, Inc., and the Commission on Collegiate Nursing Education.
	All provide standards related to curriculum and evaluation of curriculum.
	Accredited programs must ensure that their curricula meet accreditation requirements.
Licensing/certification exam requirements	Prelicensure curricula: NCLEX-PN® and NCLEX-RN® test plans and their related practice analyses.
	Graduate programs include expectations of certification examinations required for advanced practice licensure.
	The content on the test plans as well as the cognitive level at which the exams are written are equally important.
Current nursing and health care trends related to patient care and the health care environment; community and societal needs	Examples include care bundles, sepsis protocols, transitional care, adverse events in the health care environment, and improving patient outcomes.
	Addressing diversity or specific regional and societal needs in communities in which the graduates will practice.
	Gathering information from the program's stakeholders, such as the agencies that employ the school's graduates, understanding the needs of the community that the schools serves, and incorporating current trends in health care, including improving patient outcomes.
	Ensuring that the curriculum addresses the current health care environment, which requires ongoing faculty efforts to remain current in nursing practice.

not become stagnant and outdated. The meaning of the term *outdated* continues to change. The amount of data produced exceeds one's ability to assimilate it. Densen (2011), as reported in Caputi & Kavanagh (2018), noted that in 2010 medical knowledge doubled every 3.5 years; by 2020, medical knowledge is projected to double in just 73 days. A curriculum that has not been updated in 5 years may already be outdated.

Curriculum revision is an ongoing process. Once a curriculum is developed, a yearly review and revision is required based on the evaluation of student achievement of SLOs and other program evaluation metrics as well as recent initiatives in nursing and health care.

Faculty must be well versed in the entities that oversee and/or guide curricula to ensure compliance during the process of developing and implementing the curriculum. Being cognizant of these influences is important to ensure that the curriculum not only provides the means for students to achieve the SLOs but for the program to achieve program outcomes. SLOs are what individual students will achieve; program outcomes are what a group or cohort of students will achieve as a result of completing the nursing program. Program outcomes include measures such as retention rate, NCLEX pass rates, certification exam pass rates, employer satisfaction with graduates' ability to engage in current nursing practice, graduate satisfaction with the nursing program preparing them to engage in current nursing practice, and employment rate. Development of current, evidence-based SLOs that provide the educational basis for students to perform individually and as a group as measured by achievement of program SLOs and positive results on program outcomes is the hallmark of an excellent curriculum.

Scenario 4.1

The baccalaureate faculty at a major university have decided that it is time for a curriculum revision. Their curriculum is now 10 years old. Although most faculty have updated their own content, they are concerned that they have not done so in a consistent manner, resulting in curriculum drift. As the curriculum chair, you would like to outline the initial steps for faculty to consider.

Consider: What are the initial steps you will list?

LEAD THE DEVELOPMENT OF CURRICULUM AND COURSE DESIGN

Once the program SLOs and competencies are written, faculty design the courses that will be taught and the sequencing of courses across the curriculum. Faculty must keep in mind that courses in one semester build on the prerequisite courses from the previous semester. As such, all faculty are involved in developing course content that expands the student's knowledge base. This approach is superior to having each faculty member concerned with one's own content without consideration for the other courses. The idea that faculty teach in a silo without regard for previous or subsequent nursing courses is an outdated approach. For example, if in a prelicensure program an advanced medical-surgical course is taught after the maternal/child course, the advanced medical-surgical course should include case studies that involve a pregnant patient needing surgery. This helps students engage in retrieval of previously learned information and demonstrates how all the nursing information is connected.

Once the sequencing of the courses is decided, faculty develop the individual courses. Content—what students learn—is one of two major focuses of the curriculum. Initially, faculty determine what content will be taught in the program and then determine where the content will be placed in the nursing courses throughout the program.

The second major focus of the curriculum is clinical judgment. Content alone is insufficient. Students must know how to use the content, what content to use, and how to apply the content when making clinical judgments for the purpose

Table 4.3

Curriculum Models Currently Used in Nursing Programs

Curriculum Model	Brief Explanation
Traditional body systems approach: This model has been used for many years in nursing education.	Content is arranged according to specialty practice areas, such as pediatrics, mental health, and care of adults. Each course is structured around body systems and disease processes.
Concept-based curriculum (CBC): A new type of CBC began around 2007, spearheaded by Dr. Jean Giddens.	Content arranged around concepts important to the practice of nursing. Concepts are presented across health care settings, the life span, and the health-illness continuum (Giddens et al., 2020)
Using professional guidelines	Content is arranged around professional guidelines of practice. For example, master's in nursing education programs may arrange content around the NLN's *The Scope of Practice for Academic Nurse Educators* (2012).

of providing safe, quality, evidence-based, patient-centered care. Therefore, both content and thinking are leveled as students advance through the nursing courses. Bloom's taxonomy is used to demonstrate increasing levels of thinking when writing course SLOs and competencies.

Once the content and level of thinking are determined, the courses are developed. Faculty decide what content is taught in which course in the program. Most nursing programs teach simpler, easier content and lower levels of thinking in the beginning courses, then increase the complexity of content and thinking as students move through subsequent semesters. Because the purpose of the curriculum is to ensure that students are able to achieve the end-of-program SLOs and competencies, course learning outcomes and competencies are built applying the program SLOs and competencies to each course. This provides evidence that each course is structured to expand on the program SLOs across the curriculum to culminate in the program SLOs and competencies (Giddens, Caputi, & Rodgers, 2020).

Faculty determine the sequencing of courses by building on content and thinking expectations. This is often a challenge for faculty as they determine the arrangement of content within courses and the arrangement of courses within the curriculum. Faculty should apply a specific plan for making these decisions. A variety of curriculum models are used. Table 4.3 presents three common models currently used in nursing programs.

Scenario 4.2

You have taken a position as the director of a new associate degree nursing program. You are working with faculty to develop the curriculum. Faculty would like you to discuss the pros and cons of the various curriculum models available for delivery of the nursing program content.

Consider: What will you share with the faculty?

DETERMINING WHAT TO TEACH

Selecting content is the next task when developing/revising the curriculum. There are three areas to consider: content (the information students will learn), psychomotor nursing skills (those appropriate for the level of nurse the program is educating), and clinical judgment (needed at all levels of nursing education).

What is taught is a major decision for many faculty because most nursing programs tend to teach more content than is realistic for students to process. Students who are overloaded with content tend to resort to rote memorization of information rather than engaging in active learning and higher-level thinking. In prelicensure nursing curricula, many programs add additional material in the form of standardized testing, which requires students to read and review the textbooks specifically to help them pass those tests. This results in students studying two curricula, which is overwhelming and confusing for students. There is no evidence that this practice results in better prepared students.

A process for cutting content that provides general guidelines for what is and is not taught is critical to developing a successful curriculum. For example, rather than covering all diseases presented under a particular topic (such as the respiratory system or the concept of oxygenation), faculty can develop a process for deciding the top five respiratory diseases currently treated in the United States and then focus on those five. Other guidelines might relate to any additional diseases specific to the region in which the school is located and the top three medications used to treat each of the five identified diseases. Without a plan, the curriculum readily becomes "additive" and oversaturated with content.

Faculty must resist the temptation to teach volumes of information and to continually add content as nursing knowledge grows. There is no evidence for the underlying assumption that as long as content is "covered," thinking follows; that is, covering content does not in itself promote critical thinking and clinical judgment. As Benner and her colleagues found in their seminal work (Benner, Sutphen, Leonard, & Day, 2010), many faculty teach decontextualized knowledge, expecting students to know when and how to use that information in patient situations. This does not happen. If students have not been taught how to use the information in a variety of patient situations, they will not know how to use the information when called upon to do so in actual clinical situations.

Faculty then select the nursing psychomotor skills to be taught that are appropriate for the level of nurse the program is preparing. What skills will be taught in which courses is determined. How skills will be taught and evaluated must be considered. This requires the acquisition of the necessary equipment, which can include equipment for performing the psychomotor skills as well as various levels of manikins for simulated practice.

Faculty must not only teach student content and psychomotor nursing skills, but they must also teach students how to use clinical judgment to apply the content to a variety of patient situations. An ongoing problem for nursing education is an overly content-saturated curriculum. A heavy emphasis on covering as much content as possible leaves little time for students to learn and practice the application of clinical judgment to the content that they are learning. Current research indicates that students are graduating from prelicensure program not well prepared to engage in clinical judgment (Kavanagh & Szweda, 2017; Muntean, 2012). If students did not learn to think in their basic, prelicensured program, when will they learn to think? Many believe that learning to think takes time, while working in the same clinical area over a number of years. Learning to think may or may not happen in that circumstance, however. Often, nurses in one area of nursing have learned the protocols and what to do in challenging patient situations for that particular unit. When moving to a new environment, they are unable to engage in sound clinical judgment because the situations have changed and they experienced a lack of formal education on clinical judgment. Lasater, Nielsen, Stock, and Ostrogorsky (2015) found that nurses with less than 3 years of experience likely need assistance with clinical judgment as well as nurses moving to a new clinical area. Muntean (2012) reports there is ample room for improvement in clinical judgment of all frontline nursing staff and that clinical judgment can be learned at any point in the nurse's career. These research reports provide evidence that nurses at all levels of nursing education can benefit by direct, specific teaching of clinical judgment.

Masters in Nursing Education programs constitute another level of nursing education that must consider integrating teaching clinical judgment into the curriculum. If faculty did not learn clinical judgment through a formalized, systematic process in their previous nursing education programs, how will they be able to teach clinical judgment to their nursing students? Masters in Nursing Education programs should include a course on how to teach students to think; otherwise, the problem of new graduates not thinking at the required levels for safe practice will perpetuate.

The focus is now shifting to providing students opportunities to learn to process content they are learning in the way a nurse uses the information. Clinical judgment has become a major focus as faculty at all levels of nursing education engage in curriculum revision. Although faculty are accustomed to planning and teaching content and psychomotor skills, teaching clinical judgment has been very elusive. A clear, deliberated, planned, and intentional approach is what is needed to truly teach clinical judgment. Tyo and McCurry (2019) conducted an integrative review of how thinking is taught in a nursing curriculum. They discovered that there is limited evidence supporting the current methods used to teach and learn clinical judgment. They also found that using simulation or problem-based learning in the absence of a structured framework resulted in no statistically significant results; studies that used a framework to teach clinical judgment reported statistically significant increases in thinking. Therefore, nursing faculty should use a specific framework to teach and incorporate clinical judgment in a nursing program. One or two class sessions in a fundamentals course that teaches some basic information about thinking followed by teaching the nursing process is not enough. Without a planned approach to learning clinical judgment, students are expected to think and apply thinking without ever learning the clinical judgment process. Just as students require deliberate practice to perfect a psychomotor skill, so do they need that same deliberate practice applying thinking skills.

A new model for teaching clinical judgment is needed. Caputi (2016, 2018) offers a research-based model/framework with three layers.

1. The top layer of the model is Benner's (2001) Novice to Expert theory. Students begin a nursing program as a novice in nursing. They are in Benner's Novice stage, which means that they apply all the rules "as is" and are rule-based thinkers in nursing. As they complete the beginning terms, with a focus on teaching clinical judgment, faculty move the students to the next level of

thinking—advanced beginner. In this stage, they apply the rules in different ways depending on the patient context or situation. Making the transition from rule-based thinker to situation-based thinker requires that students have guided practice using the second and third layers of the model.

2. The second layer uses the four steps of Tanner's Clinical Judgment model, first published in 2006. Tanner's model provides four broad steps of the thinking the nurse uses to implement the nursing process. It is not the nursing process but rather the thinking that the nurse uses to implement the thinking process. Learning the four broad steps of clinical judgment—noticing, interpreting, responding, and evaluating—is helpful but still not enough to actually learn clinical judgment.

3. The third layer is where the details of clinical judgment are taught. The detail involves learning 19 thinking skills and strategies, or clinical judgment competencies. These are the mental skills or competencies that are required to actually apply thinking to nursing situations. These clinical judgment competencies were derived from various research-based sources including the NCLEX-RN Practice Analysis (National Council of State Boards of Nursing, 2018), the Nursing Executive Center (Berkow, Virkstis, Stewart, Aronson, & Donohue, 2011), and other nursing and education literature (Dickison et al., 2016; Levett-Jones et al., 2010). Examples of clinical judgment competencies or thinking skills include judging how much ambiguity can be tolerated in a given situation, distinguishing relevant from irrelevant information, and recognizing inconsistencies. In the first nursing course students learn all the 19 clinical judgment competencies. Once learned, students and faculty use the model/framework and its verbiage to apply clinical judgment across the entire curriculum. All faculty use the same framework as students practice clinical judgment using direct, guided practice across the curriculum to become self-regulated thinkers by the end of the program.

IMPLEMENTATION OF THE COURSE CONTENT, PSYCHOMOTOR SKILLS, AND CLINICAL JUDGMENT

Once SLOs and competencies are developed, courses are identified and sequenced across the program, course content is structured, and faculty plan the implementation of the curriculum. Questions addressed for each course include:

1. What content and psychomotor skills will be taught?
2. What thinking skills will be taught?
3. How will the content and thinking skills be taught?
4. How will the content and thinking be applied in laboratory experiences such as the clinical, skills laboratory, and simulation laboratory?
5. How will achievement of course SLOs be evaluated?

The questions in this list are best answered using a tool such as a lesson plan. Table 4.4 provides an example lesson plan. A lesson plan demonstrates a direct line of congruency among the program learning SLOs, course SLOs and competencies, unit lesson objectives, teaching/learning strategies used to deliver the lesson, and evaluation strategies. Faculty often have difficulty demonstrating this connection. The lesson plan provides this evidence. The specific unit objectives provide details about what needs to be taught.

The teaching/learning strategies provide information about how to teach the content at the appropriate level of thinking. On the lesson plan, faculty indicate

Table 4.4

Sample Lesson Plan

Program SLO	Course SLO	Competency	Unit Objectives	Teaching/Learning Strategies	Evaluation Methods
Engage in clinical judgment when making patient-centered care and other nursing decisions.	1. Demonstrate critical thinking and clinical reasoning to make patient-centered care decisions when caring for childbearing families and children.	1.1 Use critical thinking/clinical reasoning to make clinical judgments and care management decisions for the childbearing family and children to ensure accurate and safe care in all nursing actions.	**Classroom/Lab:** • Use critical thinking/clinical reasoning when making clinical judgments and management decisions to ensure accurate and safe care.	**Classroom:** • Unfolding case study, small group work assignments, then discussion to develop a concept map. • Practice items using clickers. **Clinical:** • Concept map to demonstrate links related to assessment data and nursing care with tie to clinical judgment and management decisions. • Concept map to include plans for safe care.	**Classroom:** • Unit exam: 3 application-level questions included on test blueprint. **Clinical:** • Clinical evaluation tool to include competency. • Concept map with grading rubric.
		1.2 Use critical thinking/clinical reasoning when implementing all steps of the nursing process while integrating best available evidence.	**Classroom/Lab:** • Use critical thinking/clinical reasoning to plan care using the nursing process. • Identify sources of information for best available evidence for the childbearing family and children.	**Classroom:** • Review of reliable websites for evidence-based nursing practice. • Small group work continuing the development of the concept map. • Group discussion of completed map. **Clinical:** • Concept map to include sources of best available evidence used to plan care.	**Classroom:** • Unit exam: 2 analysis-level questions included on test blueprint. **Clinical:** • Clinical evaluation tool to include competency. • Concept map with grading rubric.
		1.3 Anticipate common risks associated with the childbearing family and stable pediatric patients, and predict and manage potential complications.	**Classroom/Lab:** • Discuss types of patient data to use when planning care to decrease risks and predict and manage potential complications for the childbearing family and children.	**Classroom:** • Discuss use of informatics for data mining related to common complications and quality improvement metrics. • Small group work circling assessment data that indicate potential risks. • Group to discuss nursing interventions to prevent/manage potential complications. • Group discussion of completed map. **Clinical:** • Include on concept map specific patient data linked to potential complications with nursing interventions.	**Classroom:** • Unit exam: 1 application-level and 1 analysis-level question included on test blueprint. **Clinical:** • Clinical evaluation tool to include competency. • Concept map with grading rubric.

SLO, Student learning outcome.
© 2019, Linda Caputi, Inc. Used with permission.

the strategies used to teach content and thinking as well as any technology used to implement the curriculum through unit lessons.

Technology has become an important aspect of planning educational experiences. It is important for faculty to use technology only for an educational purpose. Never use technology just to be using technology in the absence of a clear educational reason. There are many technologies that enhance the learning experience, from virtual simulations to using an electronic medical record. These example technologies are helpful in providing a realistic, patient-situated experience. Situational learning—learning that involves a realistic health care context—strengthens the student's learning and clinical judgment (Benner et al., 2010).

Finally, the evaluation methods column of the lesson plan demonstrates how student achievement of the unit objectives will be measured. The test blueprint for development of test items links each item back to a unit objective and indicates the cognitive level of the test item. This demonstrates validity of the test—that is, the test is testing the content being taught as well as the level of thinking expected in that course as expressed through the unit objectives and course SLOs and competencies. (See Chapter 3 for an example test blueprint.) These documents demonstrate internal consistency of the curriculum; that is, all parts of the curriculum relate.

It is equally important to select appropriate clinical experiences that will demonstrate implementation of the curriculum. Clinical should be closely tied to theory. This does not necessarily mean that if care of the orthopedic patient is the topic of the theory portion of the course, students should be on an orthopedic unit for their clinical experience that week. This would be impractical in many cases. Clinical should reflect the higher levels of program and course learning outcome and their related competencies. For example, concepts such as creating a safe care environment and using sound clinical judgment reflect learning outcomes that should be part of the clinical experience each week.

Competencies for clinical nurse educators have been developed by the NLN (Shellenbarger, 2019). These competencies include:

1. Function within the Education and Health Care Environments
2. Facilitate Learning in the Health Care Environment
3. Demonstrate Effective Interpersonal Communication and Collaborative Interprofessional Relationships
4. Apply Clinical Expertise in the Health Care Environment
5. Facilitate Learner Development and Socialization
6. Implement Effective Clinical Assessment and Evaluation Strategies

Faculty can use these competencies as they plan appropriate clinical learning experiences.

Scenario 4.3

Faculty are preparing for an accreditation visit at their nursing program. They are discussing how to present to the accreditation visitors how their program is organized. They would like to demonstrate how everything they do is linked to the program learning outcomes.

Consider: What advice should you as the curriculum committee chair provide the other faculty?

DELIVERING THE CURRICULUM

The information presented in this chapter reflects educational design principles: all pieces of the curriculum are meaningful, serve a purpose, and fit together in a logical, consistent manner. All parts of the curriculum serve a purpose and are supportive of the other parts. Educational design principles, also known as instructional design, provide the basis for the total curriculum package. Faculty use educational principles, theory, and research when constructing the total curriculum package, which includes all curricular components. Educational research provides best practices that faculty can use as they implement the curriculum (Cannon & Boswell, 2016; Oermann, 2017, 2018). A review of the educational literature provides an abundance of resources.

Two important factors that faculty consider when implementing the curriculum are content taught and characteristics of students. The curriculum delivers content to address learner needs by leveling content according to the type of program: entry-level practical nursing, entry-level registered nursing, BSN completion programs, advanced practice nursing, and other graduate-level course work. Breaking down content and thinking into their component parts and determining the best approach to teaching is one aspect. For example, if the approach to teaching the content and thinking is conceptual, then theories that support conceptual learning—such as constructivist or cognitive learning theory—will be used (Giddens et al., 2020).

The other aspect to consider when selecting educational theories and research to use to deliver the curriculum is knowledge of your student characteristics. There is an array of characteristics to consider. Examples include age of the students, culture, fluency in the use of the English language, prior life experiences, prior educational experiences, and current life responsibilities. These characteristics provide data to determine whether a theory such as adult learning theory can be used to deliver the curriculum. Understanding the rationale for selecting educational principles, theories, and research to use in the design and implementation of the curriculum provides the evidence on which your approach is based (Billings & Halstead, 2016; Oermann, 2015).

Educational theory and instructional design principles continue to evolve. The main focus of face-to-face delivery of the curriculum is extended to include distance technologies. The design for the delivery of the curriculum via distance education (web-based, video, etc.) requires different considerations when the faculty and student are separated by time and distance. Faculty designing courses for delivery via distance education apply best practices that may be different than those previously used for classroom delivery (Billings & Halstead, 2016; Oermann, 2015).

An additional evolution in the design of the delivery of the curriculum relates to simulation. Designing simulation experiences requires additional strategies that may be new to faculty. It is important to use the literature when developing evidence-based strategies for delivering instruction via simulation (Jeffries, 2012, 2015).

ANALYZE RESULTS OF PROGRAM EVALUATION AND REVISE THE CURRICULUM BASED ON EVALUATION OF PROGRAM OUTCOMES, LEARNER NEEDS, SOCIETAL AND HEALTH CARE TRENDS, AND STAKEHOLDER FEEDBACK

The theoretical basis for the nursing curriculum requires ongoing faculty development. Most faculty are experts in a particular area of nursing practice and engage in ongoing continuing education related to that practice. This is critical to ensure that societal and health care trends are part of the nursing curriculum. However, education is an equally important area of expertise for faculty. Ongoing knowledge acquisition related to all aspects of curriculum development—including educational theory, practice, instructional/learning activities, and evaluation methodologies—is part of a continuing education process for nursing education faculty and administrators.

Revising the curriculum based on evaluation of program outcomes is part of the program's assessment plan. This plan is addressed in the next section.

DESIGN PROGRAM ASSESSMENT PLANS THAT PROMOTE CONTINUOUS QUALITY IMPROVEMENT; IMPLEMENT THE PROGRAM ASSESSMENT PLAN; EVALUATE THE PROGRAM ASSESSMENT PLAN

Another ongoing task for faculty is evaluating the effectiveness of the curriculum. Are the students achieving course SLOs and competencies as they move toward achieving program SLOs and competencies? Are the aggregate program outcome evaluation data at the expected levels? The evaluation phase of curriculum is often an area that receives the least amount of attention, although it is equally important as the development and implementation phases.

A systematic process is used to determine whether the program is functioning as intended. There are a number of aspects that can be included in the assessment plan:

1. student achievement of course SLOs in the classroom, laboratory, and clinical
2. achievement of expected levels on examinations such as the NCLEX and certification exams
3. retention rate
4. graduate and employer satisfaction with the educational preparation of the graduate for practice—for example, employment rates

Figure 4.1 provides an overview of the evaluation process.

Student achievement of course SLOs in the classroom is often seen as difficult to measure. However, an aid for measuring SLOs is to ensure that all information on the lesson plan is linked. The evaluation column provides the method of measuring student achievement of each unit lesson objective aligned to each course SLO and competency. The data collected from the evaluation methods are used to determine student achievement for each SLO. Box 4.1 provides an example process for measuring student learning related to course SLOs.

This same process is used for each of the course SLOs. This example is related to classroom exams, but the process is used for evaluation methods for other assignments as well. For example, a scholarly paper assignment should directly align to specific course SLOs. The paper then uses a grading rubric for the various aspects of the assignment. The grading rubric provides information about student performance linked to the course SLOs addressed by the assignment. The data are then aggregated for all students completing the assignment to determine whether the cohort has met the expected level of achievement set by faculty.

Beasley, Farmer, Ard, and Nunn-Ellison (2018) published an excellent article that provides a very clear, understandable approach to measuring student learning outcomes. In this article, the authors discuss the details of how to evaluate end-of-program student learning outcomes with both direct

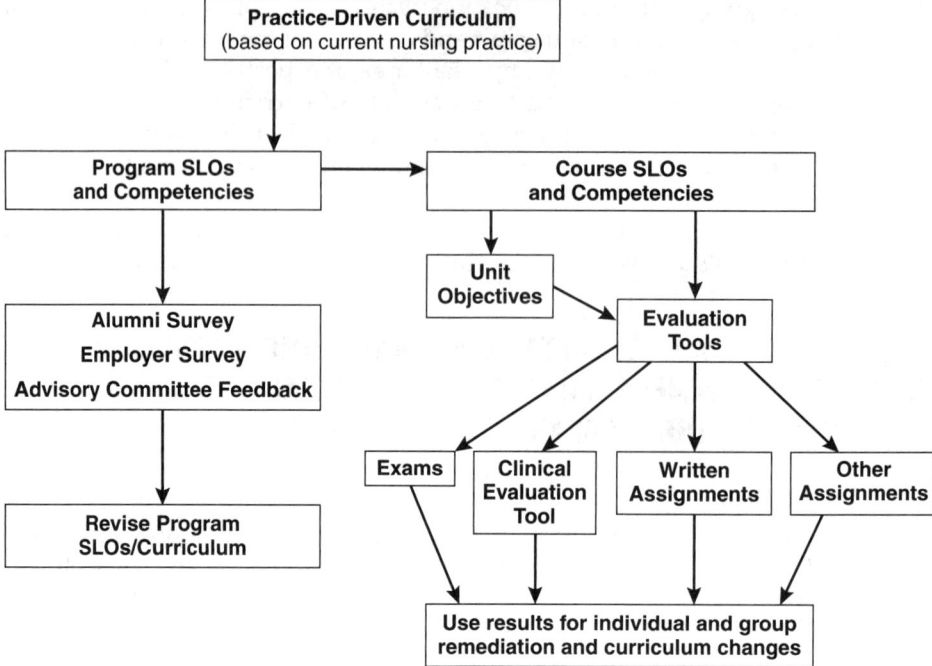

FIGURE 4.1 Curriculum Evaluation. © 2013, updated 2019, Linda Caputi, Inc. Used with permission.

BOX 4.1 Process for Evaluating Student Achievement of Course Student Learning Outcomes (SLOs)

Set an expected standard for each course SLO.

Expected Level of Achievement:
Students will score at 70% or higher on all test items related to course SLO #1.

Process:
- The test blueprint provides a link from the test item to the unit objective that is linked to the course SLO.
- All items on an exam that are linked to course SLO #1 are aggregated to determine level of performance.
- If the combined percent of all items for course SLO #1 is less than 70%, the expected level of achievement has not been met on that exam. The class needs additional instruction.
- The results of testing for items for course SLO #1 on the final exam for the course are reviewed; if students achieve 70% or higher, the level of achievement has been met for the course.
- If the expected level of achievement has not been met, faculty must determine what changes in the curriculum and/or teaching/learning strategies should be made to correct the situation. Faculty should also offer additional instruction related to SLO #1 so that current students will have the necessary information and thinking skills to progress to the next course.

© 2019, Linda Caputi, Inc. Used with permission.

and indirect assessment methods. They also discuss setting expected levels of achievement so that the evaluation data can be analyzed to determine whether SLOs have been met.

This process is also used for evaluation of clinical achievement of course SLOs. Faculty are accustomed to using clinical evaluation tools for individual student performance appraisal. However, that same data are not typically aggregated to determine whether the clinical experiences of each clinical group and of the cohort as a whole are meeting the expected levels of achievement. Aggregated data about the cohort as a whole are important to determine whether the curriculum is functioning as intended.

Scenario 4.4

You are chair of the nursing evaluation committee. The faculty believe that they do not have evidence of measuring student achievement of end-of-program learning outcomes.

Consider: What metrics can you share with faculty that they might use for this purpose?

The measures of graduate achievement of the program outcomes of NCLEX and certification exam pass rates are fairly objective. Although they are often used as a measure of program quality and achievement of program SLOs, recent practices using standardized exams as a gate for graduation from a prelicensure nursing program have confounded the NCLEX pass rates as a measure of a quality nursing program. According to Spurlock (2013), "While artificially driving up licensure pass rates may protect a program from regulatory or accreditation actions, progression policies based on high-stakes testing do nothing to improve educational program quality and divert attention from the issues that could be impacting NCLEX-RN pass rates, including poor instructional quality, disruptive or inadequate learning environments, and lack of effective learning resources" (p. 7). If schools use a commercial standardized examination as a means to graduate just those students the testing deems ready to pass the NCLEX, then the NCLEX results are not an accurate evaluation of program quality.

The percentage of students who graduate from a nursing program is an important indicator of program quality. Generally speaking, students who are accepted into a nursing program should complete the program within 150 percent of the length of the program from entry into the first nursing course. Faculty again set an expected level of achievement. The established level should reflect student characteristics, history of student retention, and expectations of the parent organization. Retention rates have become increasingly important, as the status of financial aid is affected when students do not advance or complete a program of study. Therefore, the curriculum must be constructed to be reasonable; that is, the program plan of study is designed to ensure that the credit hours and weekly clock hours required are doable for students enrolled in the program. Additionally, faculty must consider the number of hours required for out-of-class study. Credit hours are calculated as 1 credit for 3 clock hours of work. Typically, the credit hour calculation of 1 clock hour in a classroom theory session includes 2 additional clock hours of out-of-class study. Many clinical sessions are calculated at 3 clock hours of attendance for each 1 credit hour. This means that the 3 clock hours of work to earn 1 credit hour are included as part of the clinical day. Therefore, there should be no or very little out-of-clinical work expectations of the students; in so doing, students are putting in more hours than needed to earn the credit. It is critical that faculty consider all of these hours when determining the number of credit hours for each course and for the program total. Overloading students with more out-of-class work than is reasonable for the credit hours earned can result in student failure and a high attrition rate.

Nursing faculty can collaborate with community and clinical partners by gathering evaluation data about their nursing program curriculum. Collecting data to determine graduate and employer satisfaction with the nursing program and employment rates is often achieved through the use of a survey. Graduates and employers complete surveys with questions directly related to program SLOs. Both graduates and employers should evaluate the extent to which the new graduate is able to use the knowledge and thinking skills acquired through achievement of the program SLOs in their first nursing position. The value of the program SLOs should also be evaluated. That is, do the program SLOs represent what is currently important to nursing practice? Are they meeting the needs of the graduate? Do they represent societal needs and current health care trends? Only the graduates and their employers know the answers to these questions. Therefore, it is important to implement strategies resulting in a high return rate for these surveys. This often presents one of the greatest barriers to measurement of these program outcomes. Nursing programs have instituted many tactics in an attempt to experience a high return rate. Mailing surveys is perhaps the least effective strategy. Direct calls to graduates, personal visits to employers, and, more recently, the use of social media have increased return rates although requiring additional time and labor, both of which are difficult to attain, especially if the school is experiencing financial tightening. However, measuring program outcomes is not a place to decrease efforts to cut costs. If program outcomes are not measured, there is no evidence that the program is effective and no data to guide ongoing program improvement.

EVALUATE THE PROGRAM ASSESSMENT PLAN

Data that reflect the level of achievement of program SLOs and program outcomes are used to improve the nursing program. Evaluation is all about ongoing program improvement related to all aspects of the program, including the curriculum. The full range of possibilities exists depending on the results. Because a curriculum has many facets, the data must be analyzed to determine what specifically to address to improve program effectiveness. Elements of the curriculum that may be changed based on the data include:

1. student admission requirements
2. grading scale
3. sequencing of nursing courses
4. required nonnursing courses
5. teaching strategies
6. evaluation methods
7. content taught
8. integration of clinical judgment at all levels

This is not an all-inclusive list. It is obvious that data from evaluation methods are used to improve all aspects of a nursing program. Analysis of the evaluation data by faculty and nursing administration provides the basis for these improvement discussions. Any and all changes made must be evaluated to determine their effectiveness. Therefore, program evaluation is ongoing (Oermann, 2017).

LEAD THE DEVELOPMENT OF CURRICULUM DESIGN AND COURSE DESIGN; IMPLEMENT CURRICULAR REVISIONS USING APPROPRIATE CHANGE THEORIES AND STRATEGIES

The implication of the discussion in this chapter is that faculty are best positioned to be the leaders of curriculum development, implementation, evaluation, and revision. Faculty are at the forefront of the educational process and the nursing profession; therefore, they are the best prepared to engage in curriculum work. Curriculum is the responsibility of all faculty and all faculty should be informed and aware of the total curriculum and all related processes. Often, faculty work in silos, meaning that each faculty member teaches one's own course and is unable to discuss how other courses fit into the curriculum. It is important that faculty take ownership of the entire curriculum, be knowledgeable about the entire curriculum, and understand how each course contributes to the overall success of the curriculum. As faculty design the courses they teach, that design process must support the program SLOs and overall mission and purpose of the nursing program. The faculty work as a team and each individual team member contributes equally to the curriculum.

As nursing faculty engage in curriculum revision, it is important to consider the ideas of those who will be affected by the change. Applying the principles of change theory is helpful for a smooth curriculum revision.

COLLABORATE WITH COMMUNITY AND CLINICAL PARTNERS TO SUPPORT EDUCATIONAL GOALS

The curriculum is reflective of the external nursing and health care environment. As faculty work together to ensure a current, rigorous nursing program, they also work with community and clinical partners to ensure that educational outcomes are appropriate for current practice. Developing partnerships with health care agencies to ensure not just clinical placement but also an alignment of thinking related to clinical experiences is important. Additionally, in the current health care environment, nursing programs can no longer work independently. New clinical models and approaches to the curriculum must foster partnerships among faculty, students, schools, clinical agencies, staff nurses, and preceptors with the intent to align clinical learning with contemporary practice and health care needs. Nursing schools must work together "sharing resources to prepare the next generation of nurses" (Institute of Medicine, 2011, p. 174).

An additional way to collaborate with community and clinical partners is through the nursing program's advisory committee. The advisory committee consists of all parties interested in the nursing program. Members may include clinical agency staff, staff from employment agencies, graduates, current students, and nursing board representatives. The advisory committee meeting is a great place to ask for input about what is currently happening in practice as well as where the members see nursing going in the future.

SUMMARY

All nursing faculty are charged with the task of developing a curriculum that prepares students to provide safe, quality nursing care and to function within the health care environment. Developing a sound curriculum that is based on current standards, guidelines, and competencies is essential to meet that goal. Once developed, the faculty must regularly review the curriculum for currency and effectiveness and update the curriculum to facilitate ongoing program improvement. Faculty must keep current on the curriculum review/revision process to engage in this very important aspect of their scope of practice.

Practice Test Questions

1. The nursing faculty are developing competency statements for students who will participate in a clinical practicum immediately prior to graduation. Which statement is most reflective of this plan?
   A. Develop basic plans of care using the nursing process for patients with common alterations in health status.
   B. Prioritize care for assigned patients and delegate as appropriate to assistive personnel.
   C. Organize and provide all care for assigned patients.
   D. Organize and deliver care according to established priorities for patients experiencing common medical-surgical problems.

2. Faculty decide to revise an old curriculum and are developing a list of tasks. Which task should be completed first?
   A. Investigate the knowledge, skills, and attitudes needed for current nursing practice.
   B. Update the theoretical framework of the old curriculum on which to build the new curriculum.
   C. Decide whether a concept-based curriculum is best for the program.
   D. Poll the clinical agencies about their expectations of graduates.

3. A new nursing faculty is assigned to develop an adult health course as part of the curriculum revision process. Which statement best guides the faculty's development of the course?
   A. Compare the course with a similar course in a colleague's school to determine whether the content is the same.
   B. Follow the textbook when developing course outlines to ensure that all content in the book is covered.
   C. Understand that faculty are the experts; thus, the content included should be determined solely by the faculty teaching the course.
   D. Ensure that the content addresses course student learning outcomes that build on those of the prerequisite nursing courses.

4. Which statement best represents the overall purpose of a program assessment plan?
   A. Determine whether the faculty teaching strategies are effective.
   B. Determine whether the program is functioning as intended.
   C. Provide information about student characteristics as the basis for determining admission criteria.
   D. Provide data on which to develop a student retention program.

5. The director of the nursing program is chairing a meeting with the Advisory Council, consisting of clinical partners and others interested in the nursing program. Which question would be best for the director to ask of the committee members to receive input for curriculum revision?
   A. "What changes in health care do you see as important for new graduates?"
   B. "What would you like us to teach in the program?"
   C. "Are you satisfied with our graduates?"
   D. "Do the nurses on your units find the students helpful during their clinical rotations?"

6. Faculty teaching a generic baccalaureate program in nursing are considering resources to use to develop new end-of-program student learning outcomes. Which are credible resources to use for this task? Select all that apply.
   A. NLN *Outcomes and Competencies for Graduates of Baccalaureate Programs in Nursing*
   B. AACN's *Essentials of Master's Education in Nursing*
   C. QSEN competencies
   D. Listing of trends in nursing education published on *Wikipedia*
   E. Rules and regulations of the state board of nursing for nursing education programs

7. Faculty are discussing content to include in a prelicensure nursing program curriculum. Which guideline is best for faculty to adopt?
   A. Allow the faculty teaching the course to decide what content to teach.
   B. Include only content tested on the NCLEX to ensure that students are not overloaded.
   C. Teach what is covered on the standardized test that students must pass to graduate from the program.
   D. Develop a process for determining the most important content to include.

8. Faculty are discussing how to teach clinical judgment. What guideline should faculty consider?
   A. Students learn clinical judgment through experience and will become better thinkers as they progress through the program.
   B. Use a systematic, formalized plan for teaching clinical judgment using the same framework across the curriculum.
   C. Continuing the use of tactics such as asking high-level questions and employing case studies is the best approach.
   D. Nursing students are adults and are expected to be able to engage in critical thinking by the time they begin the nursing program.

9. Two nursing faculty are discussing the use of technology in nursing education. Which statement most accurately reflects best practice?
   A. "I use Facebook and Twitter because students expect faculty to use technology."
   B. "I use an electronic medical record to provide students with a realistic experience."
   C. "I prefer not to use virtual simulations because the patients are not real."
   D. "Using technology to deliver games in the classroom appeals to the new generation of students."

10. Which tool best provides evidence of internal consistency of the nursing program curriculum?
    A. Lesson plans
    B. Test blueprint
    C. Systematic plan of evaluation
    D. Model used to deliver the curriculum content

References

American Association of Colleges of Nursing. (2006). *The essentials of doctoral education for advanced nursing practice*. Washington, DC: Author.

American Association of Colleges of Nursing. (2008). *The essentials of baccalaureate education for professional nursing practice*. Washington, DC: Author.

American Association of Colleges of Nursing. (2011). *The essentials of master's education in nursing*. Washington, DC: Author.

American Nurses Association (2014). *Position statement on professional role competence*. Washington, DC: American Nurses Publishing.

Beasley, S. F., Farmer, S., Ard, N., & Nunn-Ellison, K. (2018). Systematic plan of evaluation, part I: Assessment of end-of-program student learning outcomes. *Teaching and Learning in Nursing, 13*, 3–8.

Benner, P. (2001). *From novice to expert: Excellence and power in clinical nursing practice*. Upper Saddle River, NJ: Prentice-Hall.

Benner, P., Sutphen, M., Leonard, V., & Day, L. (2010). *Educating nurses: A call for radical transformation*. San Francisco, CA: Jossey-Bass.

Berkow, S., Virkstis, K., Stewart, J., Aronson, S., & Donohue, M. (2011). Assessing individual frontline nurse critical thinking. *Journal of Nursing Administration, 41*(4), 168–171.

Billings, D. M., & Halstead, J. A. (Eds.). (2016). *Teaching in nursing: A guide for faculty* (4th ed). St. Louis, MO: Elsevier.

Cannon, S., & Boswell, C. (Eds.). (2016) *Evidence-based teaching in nursing: A foundation for educators* (2nd ed.). Sudbury, MA: Jones & Bartlett.

Caputi, L. (2010). Curriculum design and development. In L. Caputi (Ed.), *Teaching nursing: The art and science* (Vol. 1, 2nd ed., pp. 367–402). Glen Ellyn, IL: DuPage Press.

Caputi, L. (2016). The Caputi model for teaching thinking in nursing. In L. Caputi (Ed.), *Innovations in nursing education: Building the future of nursing* (Vol. 3, pp. 3–12). Washington, DC: National League for Nursing.

Caputi, L. (2018). *Think like a nurse: A handbook*. Rolling Meadows, IL: Windy City Publisher.

Caputi, L., & Kavanagh, J. M. (2018). Want your graduates to succeed? Teach them to think! *Nursing Education Perspectives, 39*(1), 2–3.

Densen, P. (2011). Challenges and opportunities facing medical education. *Transactions of the American Clinical and Climatological Association, 122*, 48–58. Retrieved from www.ncbi.nlm.nih.gov/pmc/articles/PMC3116346/

Dickison, P., Luo, X., Kim, D., Woo, A., Muntean, W., & Bergstrom, B. (2016). Assessing higher-order cognitive constructs by using an information-processing framework. *Journal of Applied Testing Technology, 17*(1), 1–19.

Emory, J. (2014). Understanding backward design to strengthen curricular models. *Nurse Educator, 39*(3), 122–125.

Giddens, J., Caputi, L., & Rodgers, B. (2020). *Mastering concept-based teaching: A guide for nurse educators*. St. Louis, MO: Elsevier.

Institute of Medicine. (2011). *The future of nursing: Leading change, advancing health*. Washington, DC: The National Academies Press.

Jeffries, P. (2012). *Simulation in nursing education: From conceptualization to evaluation* (2nd ed.). New York, NY: National League for Nursing.

Jeffries, P. (2015). *The NLN Jeffries Simulation Theory*. Philadelphia, PA: Wolters Kluwer.

Kavanagh, J. M., & Szweda, C. (2017). A crisis in competency: The strategic and ethical imperative to assessing new graduate nurses' clinical reasoning. *Nursing Education Perspectives, 38*(2), 57–62.

Lasater, K., Nielsen, A. E., Stock, M. & Ostrogorsky, T. L. (2015). Evaluating the clinical judgment of newly hired staff nurses. *The Journal of Continuing Education in Nursing, 46*(12), 563–571.

Levett-Jones, T., Hoffman, K., Dempsey, J., Jeong, S., Noble, D., Norton, C., ... Hickey, N. (2010). The "five rights" of clinical reasoning: An educational model to enhance nursing students' ability to identify and manage clinically "at risk" patients. *Nurse Education Today, 30*, 515–520.

Maine Partners in Nursing Education and Practice. (2013). Maine nurse core competencies. Retrieved from https://www.omne.org/wp-content/uploads/2016/12/ME-RN-Competencies.pdf

Muntean, W. J. (2012). Nursing clinical decision-making: A literature review. Retrieved from https://www.ncsbn.org/Clinical_Judgment_Lit_Review_Executive_Summary.pdf

National Council of State Boards of Nursing. (2018). *NCSBN research brief: Strategic practice analysis* (Vol. 71). Chicago, IL: Author.

National League for Nursing. (2010). *Outcomes and competencies for graduates of practical/vocational, diploma, associate degree, baccalaureate, master's, practice doctorate, and research doctorate programs in nursing*. New York: Author.

National League for Nursing. (2012). *The scope of practice for academic nurse educators*. New York, NY: Author.

Oermann, M. H. (2010). Curriculum revision: Making informed decisions. *Nurse Educator, 44*(1), 1.

Oermann, M. H. (2015). *Teaching in nursing and role of the educator: The complete guide to best practice in teaching, evaluation, and curriculum development*. New York, NY: Springer.

Oermann, M. H. (2017). *A systematic approach to assessment and evaluation of nursing programs*. Washington, DC: National League for Nursing.

Oermann, M. H. (2018). Wanted: Evidence to guide clinical teaching. *Nurse Educator, 43*(5), 223.

QSEN. (n.d.) QSEN competencies. Retrieved from: http://qsen.org/competencies/pre-licensure-ksas/

Shellenbarger, T. (2019). *Clinical nurse educator competencies: Creating an evidence-based practice for academic clinical nurse educators*. Philadelphia, PA: Wolters Kluwer.

Spurlock, D. (2013). The promise and peril of high-stake tests in nursing education. *Journal of Nursing Regulation, 4*(1), 4–8.

Tanner, C. (2006). Thinking like a nurse: A research-based model of clinical judgment in nursing. *Journal of Nursing Education, 45*(6), 204–211.

Tyo, M. B., & McCurry, M. K. (2019). An integrative review of clinical reasoning teaching strategies and outcome evaluation in nursing education. *Nursing Education Perspectives, 40*(1), 11–17.

Pursue Systematic Self-Evaluation and Improvement in the Academic Nurse Educator Role

Wanda Blaser Bonnel, PhD, RN, APRN, ANEF

The CNE Test Plan lists the following for the area of Pursue Systematic Self-Evaluation and Improvement in the Academic Nurse Educator Role:

Pursue Systematic Self-Evaluation and Improvement in the Academic Nurse Educator Role

A. Engage in activities that promote one's socialization to the role.

B. Maintain membership in professional organizations.

C. Participate actively in professional organizations through committee work and/or leadership roles.

D. Demonstrate a commitment to lifelong learning.

E. Participate in professional development opportunities that increase one's effectiveness in the role.

F. Manage the teaching, scholarship, and service demands as influenced by the requirements of the institutional setting

G. Use feedback gained from self, peer, learner, and administrative evaluation to improve role effectiveness.

H. Practice according to legal and ethical standards relevant to higher education and nursing education.

I. Mentor and support faculty colleagues in the role of an academic nurse educator.

J. Engage in self-reflection to improve teaching practices.

OVERVIEW

The nursing faculty role is multidimensional and requires an ongoing commitment to develop and maintain role competence (National League for Nursing [NLN], 2012a). The role requires the individual to develop and maintain competence in venues such as clinician, educator, and scholar. This competency includes components that are interactive and supportive. Ongoing quality improvement in the faculty role is a central theme uniting these components.

Quality improvement has gained emphasis with the culture of safety and quality in health care and nursing education (Institute of Medicine [IOM], 2003; Quality and Safety Education for Nurses Institute, 2019). Quality improvement serves as a basic problem-solving model that involves systematically assessing situations and implementing plans to address identified problems or gaps. It involves addressing the big picture with systems thinking, and extends to academia and faculty roles (Massey, Graham, & Short, 2007). Quality improvement models are relevant for addressing courses and programs; they are also useful for individual self-evaluation and career enhancement.

Theories, Evidence, and Tools

- Research and best evidence are key components of quality improvement. Well-developed theories and models serve as guides to help organize educator activities.
- Systems models such as the classic Donabedian (1982) model of structure, process, and outcomes are "big picture" models useful in mapping out teaching and career plans.
- The Knowles (1998) Adult Education model is a classic theory example useful in guiding teaching/learning practices.
- Boyer's scholarship (1990) and quality improvement models (Myers & Jaeger, 2012) also have relevance in career planning.

BOX 5.1 Quality Improvement

Use quality improvement (QI) approaches, such as the following:

For Self-Improvement in One's Educator Role and Career Path
- Incorporate a reflective component.
- Make time to stop and self-assess how your projects are helping you progress on your career path and what further work is needed.

Four Common Areas Benefitting from QI
- Course improvement: When developing courses and curriculum, seek feedback for needed changes for ongoing improvement.
- Classroom teaching: Maintain a healthy and inclusive learning environment.
- Clinical teaching: Work with clinical colleagues to provide a safe, quality learning environment.
- Critical incident occurrence: Be a reflective educator; use best evidence for guiding students in safe, quality patient care; learn from mistakes; help students learn from past incidents to avoid future incidents.

For Ongoing Problem Solving/QI Approaches (e.g., with a Course)
- Use problem solving for improvement: A systematic problem-solving approach is an important tool. This includes assessing or addressing the root cause analysis of a particular problem (using data to help solve problems).
- Plan and implement: Work with teams on communication and collaboration skills; engage other faculty to help solve problems (teamwork).
- Evaluate via ongoing monitoring and feedback consistent with a problem-solving model.

For Modeling QI to Students and Engaging Students in QI Opportunities
- Keep students engaged—working with clinical partners as part of the QI team, involved in quality improvement projects.
- Coach students to understand the importance of peer reviews and to gain confidence in participating in team review activities.
- Help students identify that QI is often considered learning from mistakes and involves a culture-of-safety focus to help achieve good patient and staff outcomes.

ENGAGE IN ACTIVITIES THAT PROMOTE ONE'S SOCIALIZATION TO THE ROLE

Scenario 5.1

You are assigned to help mentor two new faculty to your nursing program. You realize that you are not familiar with the new university orientation program and faculty handbook. You have not thought about approaches for helping new faculty organize professional documents to help them plan, prioritize, and highlight their projects for career progression. You have not thought about ways to help them gain networks and orientation to their assigned clinical teaching session.

Consider: What should you do next?

The academic setting presents a unique culture. Learning the role expectations and strategies to become socialized to this setting is instrumental in becoming a successful part of the culture.

- Socialization extends beyond the nursing program to include the college and larger professional community.
- Varied roles/activities within these include administrator, course leader, coach/ mentor, peer colleague, or team member.

Theories, Evidence, and Tools

- Role socialization is based, in part, on role theory, with roles based on social/ professional norms, organizational context, personal characteristics, skills, and role interpretation (Sluss, van Dick, & Thompson, 2011). Individuals take on the habits and skills needed to successfully participate in the environmental context (Blake, Ashforth, Sluss, & Saks, 2007).
- Role socialization includes spending time getting to know the academic culture. It is also guided by change and transitions models as you seek new ways, and participate in new systems as you engage in your profession.
- Strategies to support role transitions and socialization include learning your setting, getting oriented to your system, and building on the familiar. Socialization is considered an ongoing process in which individuals learn values, norms, skills, and behaviors appropriate to a social position.

Learn Your Setting

Role socialization includes gaining a good academic match initially and clarity on the type of role in which you will be employed. Questions from NLN's (2018) Healthy Work Environment Toolkit can be used to learn a setting. Sample topics from this document include:

- Role Preparation and Professional Development: Questions relate to asking about an academic setting's resources for development and how faculty gain assistance in career planning.
- Collegial Environment: Questions include asking how collegiality and community are encouraged among faculty.
- Workload and Scholarship: Questions include asking what opportunities faculty have for input into their workload responsibilities.

Get Oriented to the Setting

- Determine whether a faculty orientation process is in place and what that means to new faculty.
- Advocate for a mentor. Identify resource persons and seek opportunities to work with them.
- Learn informal and formal communication channels. Seek assistance in creating a map of faculty and staff colleagues and their roles.

MAINTAIN MEMBERSHIP IN PROFESSIONAL ORGANIZATIONS; PARTICIPATE ACTIVELY IN PROFESSIONAL ORGANIZATIONS THROUGH COMMITTEE WORK AND/OR LEADERSHIP ROLES

The multifaceted role of the nurse educator requires expertise not only in a clinical practice area but also in nursing education. Current examples include the following:

- Nursing education has experienced rapid changes over the last decade, including obvious changes such as the expanded use of simulation and online coursework. Less obvious changes relate to curriculum development, such as concept-based learning and competency-based nursing education.
- Professional organizations provide opportunities for following and addressing trends and concerns of the specialty through published reports, such as position papers. Membership in professional organizations serves as a conduit for delivery of these and many other changes.
- Membership in professional organizations is twofold: membership in clinical practice organizations and membership in nursing education organizations, such as the National League for Nursing.
- Participation and varied leadership roles can result in professional satisfaction as you give back to the organization and its causes. Networking and information exchange via these specialty organizations occur via these roles. As an active member of these associations, you are also helping to accomplish the work of the profession (Shin, 2013).

DEMONSTRATE A COMMITMENT TO LIFELONG LEARNING

Lifelong learning involves a commitment to remaining current with the rapidly changing health care world and changing needs or roles in nursing education. Efficiency is important, as this typically means commitment to regular updates on both clinical topic areas that you are teaching and best teaching/learning practices. The educator models professional behaviors for learners, including, but not limited to, involvement in professional organizations and engagement in lifelong learning activities (NLN, 2012a).

Theories, Evidence, and Tools

- Lifelong learning is central to competency in both clinical and educator practice. It is consistent with the theory of Constructivism (Taber, 2011) and constructing your learning to fit with your needs and roles.
- Benner's (1984) novice-to-expert strategies can be used as a guide to map your quality improvement plans. Useful tools to guide lifelong learning include reflective self-assessment, self-directed learning, and mapping out your learning needs.

Reflective Self-Assessment

Reflective self-assessment involves knowing yourself, including determination of what you already know related to your career role and what you still need to know (McBride, 2010).

- Reflection provides opportunity to engage one's thinking specific to experiences and to learn from these experiences, reflecting on a problem or a positive incident to consider what has been learned (Nilson, 2013).
- Self-assessment involves assessing or evaluating against some type of standard or rubric. For example, as you review this book, the NLN competencies serve as a summary of educational best practices and a type of standard. You can assess your strengths and needed areas of work related to each of the competencies.

Self-Directed Learning

Self-directed learning skills are important tools not only for faculty but students as well. Self-directed learning has a range of meanings.

- For example, in an educator course, the instructor may provide an active learning assignment or a menu of activities and let you choose those that are most relevant and meaningful. This approach allows opportunities to learn about concepts in ways that best fit your own life/career patterns.
- Tools and resources for the self-directed learner include project contracting and journaling. In a rapidly changing health care and nursing education world, these are necessary skills to maintain currency and organize vast amounts of information.

Career Mapping

Mapping out a career plan is a useful starting point for lifelong, self-directed learning. Writing out a plan can include a reflective component.

- It begins with self-assessment and involves creating a career plan or road map flowing from your personal objectives. For example, for each career objective, you might ask: What related education will I need to gain? How will I apply this learning? How will I evaluate success?
- These reflective questions serve to reinforce action steps and assist you in building your planned pathway. Mapping can be considered as orchestrating your career and evolving to a focus on outcomes (rather than a listing of activities) that can be named and described on your curriculum vitae (CV) (McBride, 2010).

PARTICIPATE IN PROFESSIONAL DEVELOPMENT OPPORTUNITIES THAT INCREASE ONE'S EFFECTIVENESS IN THE ROLE

Professional development involves strategically planning your career and considering what role development activities are needed. Efficient and effective strategies for development support not just a clinical specialty but also scholarship and teaching roles. As you stay current with trends in your clinical specialty and the best evidence about the subject matter of assigned courses you teach, you also must stay current with the best evidence for teaching and learning.

Theories, Evidence, and Tools

- The theory of adult education (Knowles, 1998) can provide direction in packaging programs that are relevant and engaging for your personal development. Tools and approaches in role development include strategic planning and use of both formal and informal educational approaches.
- Strategic planning of your education/development involves charting a course relevant to the roles you want to pursue. As you identify your career interests, you begin to identify the types of education that you will need and goals to make it happen.
- Strategic planning involves reflecting on your personal philosophy to direct goals and plans and the resources available to you, and then laying out activities to gain these as efficiently as possible.

Formal Approaches to Development

- Professional development often involves advanced education. This means making choices about what type of education program best meets your interests, needs, and the needs of your chosen academic setting.
- Common formal education approaches include the educator doctorate (EdD); the nursing practice doctorate (DNP); and the research-focused doctor of philosophy (PhD) in nursing or a related field. Certificate programs and fellowships are available as a way to document further expertise (McBride, 2010).
- Certification approaches, for those who hold a terminal degree, provide a way to document further expertise and clinical advancement. Consistent with lifelong learning, as situations or career plans change, documenting ongoing competency is key.
  - Clinical competencies can be documented via certifications such as those developed by the American Nurses Association (ANA) and other specialty organizations.
  - Educator competencies can be documented via certification with the Certified Nurse Educator® (CNE®) examination consistent with the NLN competencies (NLN, 2019).

Informal Approaches to Role Development/Continuing Education

- Attaining good resources to keep up with the rapidly changing world of health care practice and education is key to lifelong learning. Examples include reading the nursing education specialty journals and participating in journal clubs or related activities. An efficient personal system might involve staying current with several respected journals.
- Numerous nursing education journals exist, such as the NLN's *Nursing Education Perspectives*, a leader in nursing education research. Current issues in higher education are reported in journals such as the *Chronicle of Higher Education*. Clinical newsletters are valuable resources to scan for relevant clinical topics.
- Specialty organizations and clinical or academic work settings provide other educational venues for lifelong learning. For example, the NLN is a leader in providing evidence-based simulation education and care of the elderly and other vulnerable populations.
- Learning from other professionals includes seeking educational opportunities across the clinical setting or academic campus and is consistent with the move toward interprofessional education (Interprofessional Education Collaborative, 2016).

MANAGE THE TEACHING, SCHOLARSHIP, AND SERVICE DEMANDS AS INFLUENCED BY THE REQUIREMENTS OF THE INSTITUTIONAL SETTING

Expectations can be high for those in the role of educator. Some find that fulfilling multiple role expectations—typically including education, service, and research—can be very challenging and even at times unrealistic.

* Academic life and priorities will be different in an institution with a research focus versus one with a teaching focus. Approaches for balancing include being strategic and learning the realities of unique academic organizations.
* Theories, Evidence, and Tools: Boyer (1990) describes the importance of acknowledging faculty educational scholarship as well as clinical research. His classic framework for documenting educational scholarship includes teaching, application, integration, and discovery. Benner's (1984) model of novice to expert can also be relevant in documenting advancing expertise via naming and packaging scholarly products for portfolio and CV summaries.

Balancing Academic Service

Service is a common academic role along with scholarship and teaching. While scholarship and teaching are discussed in other chapters of this book, examples for balancing service roles are addressed here.

* Service is identified in multiple ways in academia. Typically, this first involves service to the academic organization and then service to the larger community, including both professional communities and community-based patient populations.
* Committee work—such as evaluation, curriculum, and student admissions/ progression committees—is often considered as service to your program/ school.
* Service to the broader community is often considered a form of giving back to the community. To gain the most value, choose service roles that mesh with authentic service work relating to your specialty interests (Cardinal, 2013).
* Service definitions may vary by types of settings. In some cases, service may be defined to include volunteer activities only.

Balancing via Role Consolidation

* Role consolidation (or combining roles), which maximizes faculty interests and minimizes workload, is considered an important practice (Bartels, 2007). For example, if opportunities to choose committee memberships exist, it is often helpful to identify a committee related to specific interests.
* When focusing on your teaching interests, it may be useful to be part of a curriculum or evaluation committee. You have a role in helping monitor or improve the quality of the academic program while gaining insights for your own course planning and evaluation practices.

Balancing with Your Team

* You and your colleague team members can also create opportunities by "dividing and conquering," for example, working together on project completion and considering multiple authors for project dissemination.
* In making the most of your team, the following questions can be helpful: Who are the key people on your team? What strategies are you using to collaborate

with clinical and academic colleagues? How do you promote a smooth working relationship and engagement with your team?

Balancing Self-Development

- Creating a manageable timeline and format that can vary by career or family responsibilities promotes balance. Balancing involves recognizing that a career is meant to last a lifetime and that all activities and projects do not need to be planned and completed all at once (McBride, 2010).
- Balancing often means assessing and planning one's activities from a big-picture focus; for example, focusing on select components of the common educator roles (teaching, service, research, and scholarship) during different semesters, years, or even different career points.
- Balance in your career can be summarized in your professional portfolio, with each chapter contributing to the whole as developed over time.

Balancing Self-Care

- Balancing involves taking care of yourself. Dealing with role stress and strain in the academic setting requires coping strategies, such as self-advocacy, to meet mutually agreed-on goals.
- Self-health promotion strategies are critical as well. As you care for yourself, you also model healthy behaviors for students and patients.

USE FEEDBACK GAINED FROM SELF, PEER, LEARNER, AND ADMINISTRATIVE EVALUATION TO IMPROVE ROLE EFFECTIVENESS

Scenario 5.2

You are just completing a course you have taught for the first time this past semester. You are concerned that there were problems with student success rates and want to improve. You have not yet reviewed students' evaluations, done a self-reflection on what worked and did not, or asked for peer feedback.

Consider: What should you do next?

Just as feedback is used in evaluating educational programs to support quality improvement, it is used to evaluate and provide guidance for faculty. Processing feedback involves being open, listening, receiving, and using the evaluation data to enhance clinical and academic activities and roles.

Theories, Evidence, and Tools

- Communication models are a major part of feedback, with listening as an active process. Feedback is considered communication of information that assists an individual in reflecting and interacting with the information to construct self-knowledge and set further goals. Feedback needs to be acknowledged and used appropriately to be effective (Bonnel, 2008; Bonnel & Boehm, 2011).
- Feedback is not considered a final grade of your work but rather a formative assessment for improving your teaching/academic efforts. It helps you gauge your accomplishments and take further responsibility for ongoing

improvement. Feedback is used to increase effectiveness in your diverse educator roles across your career. At certain career points, some types of feedback may be more important than others.

Triangulation of Methods

The concept of triangulation is an important one when considering the value of feedback. Triangulation involves gaining feedback from multiple evaluators (self, peers, learners, administration) and/or seeking use of multiple methods and approaches. Triangulation increases the credibility and validity of feedback results.

Using Student Ratings of Teaching as Feedback

- Student evaluation via class and course evaluations is a common method for acquiring feedback in academia. Gaining student feedback on courses early in the semester, rather than waiting until the end, provides time to use the feedback and make teaching or course improvements (McKeachie & Svinicki, 2013).
- Fast feedback, a best practice in classroom teaching, asks students several questions related to class learning and satisfaction. This approach provides rapid confirmation of what is working or what needs to be fixed in a classroom session. Coupled with an end-of-semester course evaluation, this helps provide a summary of both faculty strengths and further development needs.
- End-of-semester feedback from students using a standardized format is a common approach to course evaluation. While debate exists about the amount of weight to place on the final student course evaluations, in general, student ratings tend to be statistically reliable, valid, and relatively free from bias (Benton & Cashin, 2009).
- Feedback from students can be coupled with feedback from other sources and summarized in faculty yearly reviews. This process provides a quality improvement opportunity to summarize the faculty's responses to any problem areas.
- If student evaluations are troubling, it is helpful to consult with a trusted experienced colleague or mentor to deal with the disappointing student feedback. Strategies for further quality improvement can be shared by this individual (McKeachie, 2013).

Feedback from Peers and Administrators

- Peer review is described as an interactive process of providing feedback to peers based on specific criteria with the intent to promote professional growth. It is a process of communicating evaluative information that has been collected and interpreted within a comfortable environment created for this exchange (Boehm & Bonnel, 2010).
- Constructive peer feedback is often facilitated via a systematic, organized process typically incorporating a standardized rubric. Schools often have peer feedback forms available or these can be found in the literature. They provide additional data to incorporate into annual summary reviews.

Self-Assessment

- Self-assessment is a useful feedback strategy; a benefit to being an educator is always having something more to learn about oneself (McKeachie, 2013).
- Faculty can make a recording of their classroom teaching and use a rubric to self-assess classroom teaching strengths and weaknesses. This self-assessment

> **BOX 5.2 Feedback**
>
> Feedback serves as a type of formative evaluation or assessment. It is best when provided early, with room for improvement. Useful approaches are as follows:
>
> - Incorporate multiple feedback formats and synthesize these approaches to help gain a true assessment picture.
> - Optimize self-assessment and self-reflection to help identify strengths and weaknesses as well as set goals for improvement in the areas indicated (Bonnel, 2008). Use rubrics and standards as guides, such as the NLN Nurse Educator Competencies.
> - Include peer review to share thoughtful, objective critiques as a component of professional peer communication against standards such as rubrics.
> - Incorporate student evaluations or fast feedback forms across the semester for ongoing course feedback. Guide students in learning helpful professional feedback approaches.
> - Consider administrative or review committee evaluations and feedback for strengthening professional CVs or reflective portfolios.
> - Maximize technology, such as reflective e-portfolios, to help organize materials.

goes beyond the teaching content to include nonverbal and verbal cues for engaging students in learning as well as a myriad of other teaching techniques that the faculty may have used during the session. Box 5.2 provides a summary of key approaches.

PRACTICE ACCORDING TO LEGAL AND ETHICAL STANDARDS RELEVANT TO HIGHER EDUCATION AND NURSING EDUCATION

> ### Scenario 5.3
>
> You decide you need to assign a failing grade to a student in your clinical rotation. You have not addressed the evaluation rubric with students, reviewed the syllabus grading guidelines or program handbook, or talked with your faculty supervisor.
>
> *Consider:* What is wrong with this scenario.

Unique and varied ethical and legal issues are common themes throughout educational settings. Treating all individuals with respect is a key theme. In addition to teaching students important ethical and legal principles that guide their clinical practice with patients, this competency focuses on the educator's use of these tools with students in academic settings.

Theories, Evidence, and Tools

- Sound ethical and legal principles are used to develop and apply academic policies. Familiar ethical principles are relevant to academic roles as well: justice (being fair to all); autonomy (all individuals have rights); and beneficience (do no harm).
- In addition to these common principles, the classic reference from the American Association of University Professors (2009) provides a summary of specific ethical issues to which the educator should be mindful.

> **BOX 5.3 Legal/Ethical Issues**
>
> Legal and ethical considerations for educators include the following:
>
> **Use Legal/Ethical Resources/Handbooks as Faculty Guides**
> Be familiar with and communicate to students documents that guide program decisions, such as student handbooks with policies guiding appropriate professional behaviors.
>
> - Student grievance and appeal policies
> - State/national regulatory guides
> - Course syllabi and policies; student handbooks
> - Program academic integrity policies and honor codes
> - Clinical agency policies; clinical agency agreements that outline student, faculty, and agency rights and responsibilities
>
> **Keep Student Information Private**
> - Maintain the Family Educational Rights and Privacy Act of 1974 (FERPA) guidelines. This includes maintaining confidentiality related to student grades, private communications, and attendance records. These are considered confidential and are released only with appropriate consent.
>
> **Provide Students a Foundation**
> - Make students aware of policies/procedures that guide safe and reasonable practices at program admission and as appropriate throughout coursework.
> - Communicate and confirm student understanding of policies at orientation programs as appropriate throughout coursework.
> - Address both academic and clinical policies.
>
> **Help Students with Privacy and Data Management**
> - Guide students in the use of the Health Insurance Portability and Accountability Act (HIPAA), helping students keep patient information safe and private.
> - Address potential social media problems with students. Have policies regarding use of social media within clinical/classroom settings and make sure that students are familiar with them.
> - Students must understand that their behaviors on seemingly private pages are actually public and require the same professional standards of patient privacy and confidentiality (NCSBN, 2011). Appropriate policies and discussions can help prevent student missteps.
> - Legal aspects of documentation and record keeping includes addressing issues with electronic health records, such as access and not sharing passwords.

- Students have the right to due process; this includes faculty being familiar with students' rights to grievance and appeal processes. While faculty have legal guidelines in existing policies and laws, legal counsel should be sought related to student-specific legal questions or problems (Gaberson, Oermann, & Shellenbarger, 2017).
- Legal issues include student rights and responsibilities as well as faculty guidelines for achieving and promoting them. Box 5.3 further describes important resources.

Being Proactive

As outlined in Box 5.3, being familiar with and sharing with students guiding documents prior to problem development is key to promoting professional student behaviors. Best approaches to being proactive include engaging students in understanding these policies to prevent later problems. They also provide direction for how faculty can best respond if there are challenges during implementation.

Common Faculty Challenges

Common challenges in academia include being fair and consistent, promoting academic integrity, and promoting student professionalism in emerging areas, such as social networking. A proactive approach is valuable. Common issues faculty deal with relate to fairness in evaluations of classroom and clinical work.

BEING FAIR IN STUDENT EVALUATION

* Being fair and equitable in treatment of students includes having a fair grading policy for classroom, laboratory, and clinical settings. Students should receive a clear explanation about grading of assignments while providing fair evaluations in all settings. The NLN's Fair Testing Imperative in Nursing Education (2012b) emphasizes that it is crucial to be honest, clear, and objective when grading, especially in a high-stakes arena.
* Clinical settings present unique challenges and opportunities. The advent of high-technology learning labs provides valuable opportunities for a more standard clinical evaluation, such as skill check-offs with rubrics that promote student safety in actual clinical environments. It is important to establish interrater reliability for these evaluations when multiple raters evaluate students.

PROMOTING ACADEMIC INTEGRITY

Proactive strategies can also help to promote academic integrity (Clark, 2017). Proactive strategies include the following:

1. Require students to sign pledges to engage in honesty.
2. Create a safe environment that helps students feel secure enough to share actual or potential problems.
3. Identify specific assignment approaches and strategies to help avoid plagiarism.
4. Consider using tools such as a code of ethics document in post-conference discussions.
5. Engage students in developing group resources, such as a specific civility document.
6. Consider documents from national organizations, such as the student-focused National Student Nurses' Association (http://www.nsna.org/), which provide resources such as the Bill of Rights and Responsibilities for Students of Nursing.

If, after instituting proactive strategies, reactive strategies become necessary to deal with abuses of academic integrity, the following are helpful:

1. Use ongoing, clear communication, including both written and verbal formats, that document specific incidents as well as counseling efforts.
2. Define the problem behaviors and appropriate responses (e.g., student smoking is very different from intentionally being rough with a patient).
3. Align the penalty to fit the offense.
4. Use reasonable warnings with remediation opportunities.
5. Contract for improved student outcomes (including written consequences).
6. Be prepared for discussions with students about problem behaviors with documentation included, using school resources as guides for enforcing expectations.

BEING FAIR IN DEALING WITH CHALLENGING STUDENT BEHAVIORS

As faculty focus on student competency and patient safety, it can be particularly frustrating to be confronted with issues such as student tardiness or rudeness.

* Remember to focus first on proactive strategies to prevent these behaviors. Then, use fair, reasonable reactive strategies for dealing with problem behaviors.

- An example of ongoing interest is the increasing use of technology for social networking. The challenges for students to stay safe, legal, and ethical online are many. Students must understand that their behaviors on their seemingly private pages are actually public and require the same professional standards of patient privacy and confidentiality (National Council of State Boards of Nursing [NCSBN], 2011).
- Maintaining faculty professional behavior related to socialization with students is part of the professional role. Maintaining a professional student/faculty relationship involves thoughtful reflection on whether or how much socialization is appropriate. You can strive to listen to your students without getting immersed and then model a comfortable professional relationship.

MENTOR AND SUPPORT FACULTY COLLEAGUES IN THE ROLE OF AN ACADEMIC NURSE EDUCATOR

Mentoring needs and approaches vary throughout an academic career and can vary depending on the nature of the educational setting. At early career points, mentors help the new faculty to learn the ways of a program and of teaching and to help understand the unique culture of academic institutions (Slimmer, 2012). While mentoring barriers can result from limited time and faculty support for this activity, mentoring can be especially helpful in understanding this unique culture of academic institutions.

- As one progresses from novice to expert in select clinical and teaching areas, the time will arrive to help support and mentor others.
- Taking on the mentoring role involves a self-assessment about the strengths you can offer as well as seeking a good match with a mentee.

Theories, Evidence, and Tools

- A clear communication model that attends to message and sender/receiver variables is central to good mentoring. Both informal and formal mentoring concepts involve goal setting and clear communication.
- Formal mentoring moves through phases and includes key tasks and processes (Zachary, 2005). Phases such as orienting, working, and disengaging are common.
- An initial selection process for a good mentor/mentee match helps, as both mentors and mentees need to take active roles in the process.
- Reflection is considered a central concept of mentoring, with mentor and mentee reflecting together on goals for the relationship, milestones reached, or products developed.

Mentoring Toolkits

- Documents from the NLN provide guidance on mentoring (NLN, 2008, 2018). Focused to enhance faculty career development as well as promote healthy work environments, these documents describe mentoring programs as early-, mid-, and late-career programs. A series of questions and resources guide mentoring assessments and practices at varied career points. Select approaches are noted in Box 5.4.

Box 5.4 Mentoring

Mentoring is considered a guided experience that facilitates development and seeks positive outcomes as described by the profession or context:
- Mentoring varies with your point on a career continuum (NLN, 2008).
- A spectrum of mentoring exists from formal program to informal situational mentoring.

Useful tools in mentoring include:
- Skillful listening; asking important questions
- Affirming and challenging (feedback); creating accountability (Bonnel, Smith, & Hober, 2018)
- Guided reflective opportunities, such as journaling and reflective logs
- Helping to network and develop professional relationships (this can include local as well as broader professional interactions)
- Guiding toward resources such as needed textbooks, journals, and educational programming
- Helping the mentee put together a plan with priorities determined by the mentee's self-assessment and importance of needs

---

- Mentoring can involve diverse models—including dyad, functional, and group approaches—to support mentees into a professional culture (Kashiwagi, Varkey, & Cook, 2013).
- Mentoring can also be at a distance, using technologies to promote student, colleague, and faculty mentoring communications.
- A synthesis of research literature found that mentoring had a positive impact on career, attitude, relationships, and motivational outcomes (Nowell, Norris, Mrklas, & White, 2016). The value of mentoring to the profession as a whole is also described (Shin, 2013).

ENGAGE IN SELF-REFLECTION TO IMPROVE TEACHING PRACTICES

Scenario 5.4

You are planning to work with your assigned mentor to organize your first promotion packet. You realize that you do not know your organization's specific policies and procedures for promotion; the process and calendar to be followed; the types of documentation needed by a designated review committee; or the criteria to be used to assess such a packet.

Consider: What should you do next?

Self-reflection while advancing through a career trajectory keeps the nurse educator focused on the most important aspect of the life of an educator—that of improving teaching practices. Just as career advancement for a nurse in clinical practice is all about improving patient outcomes, so is career advancement for a nurse educator all about improving teaching and learning. The academic culture broadly appreciates a focus on documenting progress in education, service, and scholarship activities. The CV and portfolio provide reflective documentation opportunities.

Theories, Evidence, and Tools

- The Scholarship of Teaching and Learning model (Boyer, 1990) provides direction for ongoing quality improvement related to your career planning and documenting via CVs and portfolios. Naming what you do in your professional educator role can be clarified by Boyer's four scholarly categories: education, practice, integration, and discovery. Selected tools and approaches to guide progression, change, and transitions include seeking a good academic fit and documentation via a CV and portfolio.

Seek a Good Academic Fit

Gaining clarity on a particular school's academic system provides a good start for matching personal interests with career planning (Penn, Wilson, & Rosseter, 2008). Schools with a specific research mission often require different faculty competencies or processes than those for faculty who want to focus on teaching and service (Bartels, 2007). Seek a good academic fit and faculty appointment type that fit with your career goals.

- This involves knowing about types of academic settings and faculty appointments as well as the concepts of tenure and promotion. Ask questions such as (1) Will I be adjunct faculty, clinical faculty, or research faculty? and (2) Will my role be in a research-intensive or teaching-intensive university?
- Research-intensive institutions focus more on research products while academic-intensive institutions focus more on educational scholarship. Finding a good match with your interests and the institution's needs is key (McBride, 2010).
- A good academic fit involves learning about a program's system for promotion and tenure. You will begin with questions such as (1) What type of appointment will I have? and (2) What type of education is required for different appointments?
- You will seek orientation to the organization's policies and procedures related to tenure:
  1. The process and calendar to be followed
  2. The types of documentation needed by the tenure committee
  3. The criteria to be used to assess the tenure packet
  4. The process for weighting the types of faculty activities/outcomes (Diamond, 2002)

You will plan to learn about faculty development opportunities provided for selected roles. Finally, develop a CV and, typically, a portfolio that flows from and matches your plan.

Developing a Curriculum Vitae and Portfolio

Career progression is much about setting career goals and building your CV as the semesters and years advance. Understanding your school's mission, job descriptions, and promotion/tenure guidelines facilitate your professional development and progression over time.

- Your CV may be referred to as an enhanced résumé. It provides a detailed summary used to document progression of professional experiences. The CV involves clearly naming and describing to others what you do and your areas of interest (McBride, 2010). This is a professional document that does not include personal or family information.
- CV components can relate to the traditional teaching, research, and service roles or Boyer's (1990) expanded criteria. Building a CV involves the inclusion of professional areas you want to emphasize and demonstrating progress in your selected roles. McBride (2010) describes the value of documenting transitions or advancement from the home stage to the broader health care professional field.

Naming your products and activities as you progress from novice to expert in an area shows your professional growth.

A portfolio is a collection of writings and documents that summarize your work and experiences. This can be as simple as a notebook documenting your accomplishments and showing samples of your work.

- Portfolio development complements your CV and highlights self-directed, lifelong learning. Portfolios can help document learning and showcase your teaching/learning process and outcomes. Benefits of portfolios include helping to document progress in multiple career components (both in clinical and educator contexts) over time.
- With varied approaches for structuring portfolios, key concepts include communication about what you do and reflection on what you do. An example is describing a course that you teach and then reflecting on the course successes and challenges. This portfolio component tells your story of course development and how you shared this professionally with others as part of professional development.
- As you create your personal portfolio, each component contributes to the whole. While different career points in time focus on different areas, the complete portfolio shows the big picture of your career, helping to define what you do as a professional.

SUMMARY

Quality improvement as a nurse educator includes not just staying busy with activities but also demonstrating products and progression in the various academic roles. Gaining a vision of what an academic career looks like and finding a good academic setting match for your interests and skills provides a good beginning to role socialization. Assessing one's strengths and desires, seeking education and mentoring opportunities for lifelong learning, seeking and using feedback, and learning to balance the various roles of an academic nurse educator provide a firm basis for ongoing improvement in career and program quality.

Practice Test Questions

1. The nurse educator is meeting with new nursing students. Which strategy will the faculty consider as a priority to promote academic integrity?
   A. Review the course calendar for exam deadlines.
   B. Review the course syllabus for academic integrity guidelines.
   C. Require students to purchase antiplagiarism computer devices.
   D. Require students to work as partners for test taking.

2. Which statement by a faculty member concerning career balance suggests the need for further mentoring?
   A. "I am using what I am learning from my evaluation committee work to help develop my new nursing course."
   B. "I am working with a physical therapy colleague to write a paper about functional assessment."
   C. "Often, I use the same project for both a presentation and then a publication."
   D. "My personal goal is to submit three manuscripts I write this month and then three next month."

3. Following an educational session on legal and ethical issues, the nurse educator is concerned to hear a colleague make which statement?
   A. "Syllabus development needs to include a focus on grade policies and policies on cheating."
   B. "Problem solving for best solutions is a common approach to a legal or ethical issue."
   C. "Students should be required to share a copy of a patient's clinical record with colleagues at post-conference to help validate their clinical experiences."
   D. "Nursing faculty should have tools and guidelines to assist and teach ethical decision-making."

4. The nurse educator wonders whether a student has plagiarized large parts of a formal paper. The educator is especially concerned when the educator hears a student make which statement?
   A. "I did my best to follow what the school handbook says on plagiarism."
   B. "I attended the orientation session students received on descriptions and examples of plagiarism."
   C. "I was happy that technology allowed me easy opportunities to copy key sentences into my paper."
   D. "I signed a pledge that says I will follow the honesty policies of the school."

5. The nurse educator is co-teaching a course and wants to consider continuous quality improvement (CQI) in course implementation. The nurse educator is concerned upon hearing a fellow faculty member make which statement?
   A. "I will seek feedback throughout the course I am teaching."
   B. "I will put priority on the one final student evaluation at semester end."
   C. "I will consider both my content and teaching expertise as I self-evaluate."
   D. "I can use feedback from multiple sources, such as peer review and self-reflection, to make changes and improve the quality of the next offering of the course."

6. Seeking a new faculty position, the nurse educator applies to a large university and wants to confirm that the program is a good fit for the nurse educator's interests and career plans. A colleague expresses concern upon hearing the applicant make which statement?
   A. "I want to have an active role in processes and policy decisions in my program."
   B. "I want to be part of not just the nursing program but the larger university academic setting."
   C. "I understand different types of programs (such as community colleges and universities) have different missions and might indicate different faculty roles."
   D. "I think I would have more opportunities and support for a nursing research career at the local community college."

7. The nurse educator is updating the CV. A faculty colleague expresses concerns if the educator makes which statement?
   A. "When I document the many projects that I have completed, it just feels like I am bragging."
   B. "Building a CV and portfolio involves planning for areas of emphasis and showing progression in my selected roles."
   C. "I want to document my project advancement from my local program to the broader professional nursing field and organizations."
   D. "Naming and documenting my products and activities as I progress from novice to expert in an area shows my professional growth."

8. The nurse educator is seeking promotion at a major university. The educator's mentor expresses concerns when hearing that the mentee plans include which of the following?
   A. Seeking orientation to the organization's policies and procedures for promotion
   B. Seeking an extension of the calendar deadline so that the educator can work harder on self-documentation
   C. Considering the types of documentation outlined by the review committee
   D. Addressing the criteria and criteria weighting to be used to assess the promotion packet

9. The nurse educator has concerns upon hearing a new faculty colleague make which comment about professional organization membership?
   A. "I am trying to build my résumé and adding a membership to a professional organization will look good."
   B. "I appreciate how national organizations help me stay current on the changing needs of society and might help generate ideas for curriculum change."
   C. "I like how some professional organizations provide a national voice for nurse educators on important professional issues."
   D. "I use position papers and summaries from the national organizations to stay aware of changing issues in our profession."

10. The nurse educator is asked to assist in developing a new faculty orientation program. Which statement from a co-faculty member would be of concern?
    A. "We should find value in addressing Benner's novice-to-expert model."
    B. "We can ask new faculty to talk with assigned mentors about the challenges they are finding."
    C. "We should emphasize our program policies rather than the broader university policies."
    D. "We should include time for orientation to the clinical unit faculty will be working on."

11. The nurse educator has concerns about the mentoring that a faculty colleague has received upon hearing him make which statement?
    A. "I want to seek multiple mentors for varied career interests and academic needs."
    B. "My mentor has outlined a developmental plan for me."
    C. "I will use technology to help organize my scholarly materials."
    D. "I am using a writing coach to increase my professional publication skills."

12. The nurse educator is working as a direct supervisor to a new faculty member who has shared concerns of potentially having to fail a student. Which comment from the faculty member causes the nurse educator concern?
    A. "I have documented the conferences I had with this student."
    B. "The information about failing will be a surprise to my student since he has not been engaged during our conversations."
    C. "I have met regularly with the student to provide feedback and suggest improvements."
    D. "I have reviewed the course syllabus and program handbook with my clinical students."

References

American Association of University Professors. (2009). Statement on professional ethics. Retrieved from https://www.aaup.org/report/statement-professional-ethics

Bartels, J. (2007). Preparing nursing faculty for baccalaureate level and graduate level nursing programs: Role preparation for the academy. *Journal of Nursing Education, 46*(4), 154–158.

Benner, P. (1984). *From novice to expert: Excellence and power in clinical nursing practice.* Menlo Park, CA: Addison-Wesley.

Benton, S. & Cashin, W. (2009). Student ratings of teaching: A summary of research and literature. The IDEA Center. Retrieved from https://www.ideaedu.org/Portals/0/Uploads/Documents/IDEA%20Papers/IDEA%20Papers/PaperIDEA_50.pdf

Blake, A., Ashforth, B., Sluss, D., & Saks, A. (2007). Socialization tactics, proactive behavior, and newcomer learning: Integrating socialization models. *Journal of Vocational Behavior, 70*(7), 447–462.

Boehm, H., & Bonnel, W. (2010). The use of peer review in nursing education and clinical practice. *Journal for Nurses in Staff Development, 26*(3), 108–115.

Bonnel, W. (2008). Improving feedback to students in online courses. *Nursing Education Perspectives, 29*(5), 290–294.

Bonnel, W., & Boehm, H. (2011). Faculty practices in providing online course feedback. *Journal of Continuing Nursing Education, 42*(11), 503–509.

Bonnel, W., Smith, K., & Hober, C. (2018). *Teaching with technologies in nursing and health professions: Strategies for engagement, quality, and safety* (2nd ed.). New York, NY: Springer.

Boyer, E. L. (1990). *Scholarship reconsidered: Priorities of the professoriate.* Princeton, NJ: The Carnegie Foundation for the Advancement of Teaching.

Cardinal, B. (2013). Service vs. serve-us: What will your legacy be? *Journal of Physical Education, Recreation & Dance, 84*(5), 4–6.

Clark, C. (2017). An evidence-based approach to integrate civility, professionalism, and ethical practice into nursing curricula. *Nurse Educator, 42*(3), 120–126.

Diamond, R. (2002). *Serving on promotion, tenures, and faculty review committees: A faculty guide.* Bolton, MA: Anker Publishing Company.

Donabedian, A. (1982). *The criteria and standards of quality.* Ann Arbor, MI: Health Administration Press.

Gaberson, K., Oermann, M., & Shellenbarger, T. (2017). *Clinical teaching strategies in nursing* (3rd ed.). New York, NY: Springer Publishing.

Institute of Medicine. (2003). *Health professions education: A bridge to quality.* Washington, DC: The National Academies Press.

Interprofessional Education Collaborative. (2016). *Core competencies for interprofessional collaborative practice: 2016 Update.* Washington, DC: Retrieved from https://www.tamhsc.edu/ipe/research/ipec-2016-core-competencies.pdf

Kashiwagi, D., Varkey, P., & Cook, D. (2013). Mentoring programs for physicians in academic medicine: A systematic review. *Academic Medicine, 88*(7), 1029–1037.

Knowles, M. (1998). *The adult learner: The definitive classic in adult education and human resource development* (5th ed.). Houston, TX: Gulf Publishing.

Massey, W., Graham, S., & Short, P. (2007). *Academic quality work: A handbook for improvement.* Bolton, MA: Anker Publishing Company.

McKeachie, W. J., & Svinicki, G. (2013). *McKeachie's teaching tips: Strategies, research, and theory for college and university teachers* (13th ed.). Belmont, CA: Wadsworth Publishing.

McBride, A. (2010). *The growth and development of nurse leaders.* New York, NY: Springer.

Myers, J., & Jaeger, J. (2012). Faculty development in quality improvement: Crossing the educational chasm. *American Journal of Medical Quality, 27*(2), 96–97.

National Council of State Boards of Nursing. (2011). White paper: A nurse's guide to the use of social media. Retrieved from https://www.ncsbn.org/Social_Media.pdf

National League for Nursing (2008). The mentoring of nursing faculty toolkit. Retrieved from http://www.nln.org/docs/default-source/recognition-programs/toolkit.pdf?sfvrsn=4

National League for Nursing (2012a). *The scope of practice for academic nurse educators.* New York, NY: National League for Nursing.

National League for Nursing. (2012b). The fair testing imperative in nursing education: A living document. Retrieved from http://www.nln.org/docs/default-source/about/nln-vision-series-%28position-statements%29/nlnvision_4.pdf

National League for Nursing. (2019). Certified nurse educator candidate handbook, 2019. Retrieved from http://www.nln.org/docs/default-source/default-document-library/cne-handbook-july-2019-rev.pdf?sfvrsn=0

National League for Nursing. (2018). Healthful Work Environment Toolkit. Retrieved from http://www.nln.org/docs/default-source/professional-development-programs/healthful-work-environment-toolkit.pdf?sfvrsn=20

Nilson, L. (2013). *Creating self-regulated learners: Strategies to strengthen students' self-awareness and learning skills.* Herndon, VA: Stylus Publishing.

Nowell, L., Norris, J., Mrklas, K., & White, D. (2016). Mixed methods systematic review exploring mentorship outcomes in nursing academia. *Journal of Advanced Nursing, 73*(3), 527–544.

Penn, B., Wilson, L., & Rosseter, R. (2008). Transitioning from nursing practice to a teaching role. *Online Journal of Issues in Nursing, 13*(3). Retrieved from http://ojin.nursingworld.org/MainMenuCategories/ANAMarketplace/ANAPeriodicals/OJIN/TableofContents/vol132008/No3Sept08/NursingPracticetoNursingEducation.aspx

Quality and Safety Education for Nurses Institute. (2019). QSEN competencies. Retrieved from http://qsen.org/competencies/pre-licensure-ksas/

Shin, L. (2013). Current issues in nursing associations. In D. Mason, J. Leavitt, & M. Chaffee. *Policy and politics in nursing and healthcare* (6th ed., pp. 602–608). St. Louis, MO: Elsevier.

Slimmer, L, (2012). A teaching mentorship program to facilitate excellence in teaching and learning. *Journal of Professional Nursing, 28*(3), 182–185.

Sluss, D. M., van Dick, R., & Thompson, B. S. (2011). Role theory in organizations: A relational perspective. In S. Zedeck (Ed.), *APA handbook of industrial and organizational psychology. Building and developing the organization* (Vol. 1, pp. 505–534). Washington, DC: American Psychological Association.

Taber, K. S. (2011). Constructivism as educational theory: Contingency in learning, and optimally guided instruction. In J. Hassaskhah (Ed.). *Educational Theory.* United Kingdom Edition: Nova.

Zachary, L. J. (2005). *Creating a mentoring culture. The organization's guide.* San Francisco, CA: Jossey-Bass.

6

Function as a Change Agent and Leader

Theresa M. "Terry" Valiga, EdD, RN, CNE, FAAN, ANEF

The CNE Test Plan lists the following for the area of Function as a Change Agent and Leader:

Function as a Change Agent and Leader

1. Function as a change agent and leader in this manner:
- Model cultural sensitivity when advocating for change
- Evaluate organizational effectiveness in nursing education

2. Enhance the visibility of nursing and its contributions by providing leadership in the:
- nursing program
- parent institution
- local community
- state or region

3. Participate in interdisciplinary efforts to address health care and educational needs:
- within the institution
- locally
- regionally

4. Implement strategies for change within the:
- nursing program
- institution
- local community

5. Develop leadership skills in others to shape and implement change.

6. Adapt to changes created by external factors.

7. Create a culture for change within the:
- nursing program
- institution

8. Advocate for nursing, nursing education, and higher education in the political arena.

The Certification Test Development Committee of the National League for Nursing (NLN) Certification Commission (2012, p. 19) asserts that "nurse educators function as change agents and leaders to create a preferred future for nursing education and nursing practice. To function effectively as a change agent and leader, the nurse educator:

- models cultural sensitivity when advocating for change
- integrates a long-term, innovative, and creative perspective into the nurse educator role
- participates in interdisciplinary efforts to address health care and educational needs locally, regionally, nationally, or internationally

- evaluates organizational effectiveness in nursing education
- implements strategies for organizational change
- adapts to changes created by external factors
- provides leadership in the parent institution as well as in the nursing program to enhance the visibility of nursing and its contributions to the academic community
- promotes innovative practices in educational environments
- develops leadership skills to shape and implement change"

It is clear from this charge that taking on the responsibility of leadership and functioning as a change agent in and for nursing education is something that lies within each faculty member and is not limited only to those who hold formal administrative positions in an organization. Too often, faculty look to department chairs, program directors, or deans to formulate a vision for program development in a particular school. The reality, however, is that faculty also must function as leaders who help articulate and then shape that vision—that preferred future—for the school. Likewise, faculty often look to boards of national organizations to determine standards related to education and feel that they have no role in determining what excellence in nursing education looks like. Again, the reality is that faculty are the leaders and change agents who define excellence, identify the support and resources needed to achieve excellence, and lead change initiatives designed to continually pursue that goal. Leadership, therefore, is not something that belongs only to individuals in formal positions of authority. But what is leadership? And how is it the same as, and different from, management?

FUNCTION AS A CHANGE AGENT AND LEADER; ENHANCE THE VISIBILITY OF NURSING AND ITS CONTRIBUTIONS BY PROVIDING LEADERSHIP

Grossman and Valiga (2017) acknowledge that "defining just what leadership is, who leaders are, what leaders do, and how leadership is different from management—a phenomenon with which it often is confused—is no easy task" (p. 2). These authors assert that leadership and management are different (Table 6.1):

Table 6.1

Comparison of Leaders and Managers

Leader	Manager
A role for any individual in an organization	A role assigned to an individual by virtue of the person's position in an organization
Collaborates with others to identify and work toward goals that will create more positive environments and advance excellence	Establishes or reinforces processes to meet goals set by the organization
Appreciates that visions are realized over time	Strives to achieve goals in the most efficient and cost-effective manner possible
Strives for excellence	Limits new initiatives in order to get the work done and on time
Gains power through what the individual knows, trusting relationships, and credibility	Gains power through the individual's ability to reward or punish others and to control resources

leadership can be learned, and each of us can and should be a leader. These concepts are congruent with the competency that the NLN has outlined for nurse educators.

Management is a function carried out by individuals in formal positions of authority. By virtue of their position, such individuals are expected to ensure that their subordinates work to fulfill the goals of the organization, are expected to have an eye on "the bottom line" and not necessarily on the horizon, and work to minimize disruption so that tasks can be accomplished in a timely and efficient manner. Their power comes from their position and may be demonstrated through reward (e.g., preferred teaching assignments) and/or punishment (e.g., classes scheduled late on Friday afternoons).

Leadership, in contrast, is a function carried out by any number of individuals in an organization. Leaders have their eye on a long-term vision of excellence, a vision that they articulate clearly and with passion, and which serves to entice others to join efforts to achieve it. Leaders, therefore, arise from the group and are given power to influence that group by virtue of their knowledge, credibility, passion, and ability to motivate others. They work collaboratively with followers to achieve a goal that is created and shared by all and not merely imposed by the organization.

Leaders and Followers

Many often bristle at the notion of themselves or others being thought of as followers. In essence, however, there can be no leaders if there are no followers. Effective followers are not sheep who follow blindly, however. Instead, they are thinking, passionate, motivated individuals who participate actively in making change happen and shaping a new, preferred future.

Essentially, effective followers have many of the same characteristics as leaders (Table 6.2). They are forward-looking, question and challenge the status quo, are comfortable with change, are willing to take risks, are actively involved, and think critically about and challenge ideas that are presented to determine the best possible decision or course of action.

Table 6.2

Selected Characteristics of Leaders and Effective Followers

Leaders	Followers
Think critically	Look forward with an "eye on the horizon"
Question and challenge the status quo	Comfortable with change
Willing to take risks	Actively involved
Communicate effectively	Strive for excellence
Build positive, reciprocal relationships	Offer ideas for improvement
Recognize and build on strengths of others	Comfortable with uncertainty and ambiguity
Work collaboratively with others	Well-informed with broad perspective

Followers with these characteristics often assume a leadership role when needed to keep the group moving toward its vision, and they build positive, reciprocal relationships with the entire team, including the recognized leader. Followers, therefore, are critical for change to occur, and they are essential if leaders are to help shape a preferred future.

Scenario 6.1

Marcus is an associate professor in a school of nursing housed in a comprehensive institution. He is an experienced faculty member on a nontenure-earning track whose workload is heavily weighted toward teaching, though he also is expected to engage in scholarly activities and provide service to the school and within the profession. He is passionate about teaching and wants that aspect of the school's tripartite mission to be acknowledged for its excellence. He believes that achieving designation as an NLN Center of Excellence (COE) in Nursing Education is a way to do that. Marcus talks with other faculty whom he knows share his passion; together, they outline a plan to move forward toward achieving COE designation. He leads his colleagues in developing a proposal that includes the COE category to be pursued, examples of how the criteria in this category are being met, a timeline for completing the COE application, the financial and human resources that would be needed to prepare and submit that application, and individuals who have agreed to serve on the team that will lead the COE initiative. That proposal is presented to and discussed with the dean, who offers support and commits the needed financial resources. It is then presented to the entire faculty, who conduct a discussion of the benefits of COE designation and ways in which all faculty will participate in the process.

Consider:
1. In what ways has Marcus demonstrated leadership?
2. How has he engaged followers?
3. What kind of relationships with other members of the school's community will Marcus and the COE team need to develop and sustain to ensure that evidence is provided in the application to document how the school has met each COE criterion in the chosen category?
4. How can Marcus take full advantage of the talents of all team members so that the leadership abilities of each are maximized and strengthened?

Managers and Administrators as Leaders

As noted, every faculty member has the opportunity—and responsibility—to take on the role of leader when needed to continually improve nursing education. Fortunately, many faculty members do take on this responsibility. However, leadership in an organization also is provided by faculty who hold positions such as course coordinators, level coordinators, or committee chairs, as well as by individuals who are in formal positions of authority: deans, chairpersons, directors, and so on.

Leaders, as noted earlier, often emerge from and are followed by members of a group because of the vision they espouse. Individuals in formal positions of authority, on the other hand, typically are appointed by some external individual or group (e.g., Vice President for Academic Affairs, Provost). Such appointments reflect support of the individual's vision for the school/program, ability to help a group/organization grow and evolve, and ability to lead change. Thus, they have many of the same characteristics that have been described for leaders.

Deans and directors are expected to collaborate with faculty to outline goals for the school/program and formulate plans to reach those goals. Some potential goals are increasing the number of qualified students who apply for admission, increasing graduation rates, improving program outcomes, offering programs in innovative formats, increasing the number of faculty prepared for doctorates, increasing the amount of external grant funds received, offering new graduate-level specialties, or enhancing the influence of the school/program within the parent institution. These are examples of important goals that require extensive planning and resources to achieve and that are met through collaborative efforts among administrators, faculty, clinical partners, and other offices/departments within the institution.

Administrators have the responsibility for ensuring that the work of the school/program is aligned with that of the parent institution; they often are called upon to provide evidence of such congruence. They have overall responsibility for developing and managing the budget for the school/program, often are the final decision-makers related to faculty appointments, serve as spokespersons for the school/program, and are expected to provide input to committees and/or higher-level administrators regarding faculty promotion or tenure decisions.

Faculty aspiring to an administrative role, therefore, need to develop strong management skills as well as skills of leadership. Additionally, they need to learn to effectively balance those responsibilities. The dean/director who puts too much emphasis on management may contribute to the evolution of a highly efficient system with a "positive bottom line" but also a system that is unwilling to change for fear of introducing uncertainties, raising the possibility of failure, and jeopardizing efficient operations. On the other hand, the dean/director who puts too much emphasis on leadership may contribute to the evolution of a system that is in constant flux, does not stay within its budget, has no clear sense of direction, and does not meet expectations set by upper administration. Therefore, it is important that individuals in formal positions of authority know when to "push" change and innovation and when to move toward change in a cautious, deliberate manner.

IMPLEMENT STRATEGIES FOR CHANGE; DEVELOP LEADERSHIP SKILLS IN OTHERS TO SHAPE AND IMPLEMENT CHANGE

As noted earlier, both leaders and followers are driven toward excellence and a preferred future, and administrators/managers typically value excellence as well. To reach such goals, it must be understood that change is essential, that members of the organization must be challenged to think in new ways, and that all members of the school are supported as they encounter uncertainties on the journey. All administrators and faculty understand that change is a "messy" process. Although experts have outlined phases of change potentially suggesting that all that is needed is to follow a prescribed path and all will be well, the truth is that change can be quite threatening to many individuals. Feeling threatened may prompt individuals to act in ways that seem to "stall" or provide "roadblocks" to achieving the new goal.

The effective leader and change agent (see Table 6.2) recognizes that attention must be paid to the individuals in the group—their backgrounds, past experiences with change, self-confidence, comfort with ambiguity and uncertainty, cultural practices, and sense of vulnerability (e.g., when faculty members who are approaching a tenure or promotion review seem unwilling to openly oppose ideas presented by members of the committee who will review their dossiers). Attention also must be paid to the group as a whole, taking into consideration the group's past experiences with change and its aftermath, the degree of collegiality and civility (Clark, 2017) in the group, the group's culture regarding decision-making, and the resources available to support change efforts.

Motivating and leading a group to change involves the stages outlined by the classic work of Lewin (1951). Although this theory was proposed nearly 70 years ago, it still has relevance and is still useful to leaders. Lewin noted that the first phase of change is *unfreezing*, during which members of the group prepare for change. Once the need for change has been accepted, the phase of *moving* occurs in which the design and implementation of the change itself takes place. Finally, the phase of *refreezing* occurs as the change is integrated into the system and becomes part of the new norm.

The perspective on change suggested by Lewin (1951) is one of evolution; a change is planned, gradually introduced, and may take an extended period of time before it becomes fully integrated into the system and culture of the organization or group. In contrast, recent literature (Christensen, Raynor, & McDonald, 2015) addresses a more revolutionary perspective on change. Disruptive innovations or technologies serve to turn systems upside-down rather quickly, ideas are adopted rapidly, and groups or organizations strive to be "on the cutting edge" in the field. Such change may be referred to as *transformative*, in which key aspects of the organization are changed dramatically: its *structure* (i.e., who reports to whom, the names and functions of departments or subunits), its *processes* (i.e., how decisions are made), and its *culture* (i.e., how things are viewed, what is valued and rewarded).

The nursing education leader needs to be comfortable with both evolutionary and revolutionary change. For example, when proposing a new curriculum

---

Scenario 6.2

Janice is an assistant professor in the school of nursing at the local university. She is an accomplished clinician and has solid theoretical and practical grounding in teaching and learning. In her own clinical practice and when she is on clinical units with students, Janice becomes acutely aware of the many opportunities that nurses have to influence change in how they practice on their unit and how, time and again, they fail to take advantage of those opportunities. She talks with these nurses and learns that they do not think they have the right to suggest changes because they are not the manager or supervisor, they are not certain of what changes to propose, and they are not confident that they have the communication skills, credibility, or strength to try to make a difference.

As a member of the school's curriculum committee for the undergraduate program, Janice wants to ensure that the students in her program graduate with the knowledge, skills, and confidence needed to function as leaders in their practice settings and lead change that will enhance the quality of care provided to patients and their families. Her committee colleagues, however, do not see this as an urgent focus and believe that more time needs to be spent on covering content.

Consider:
1. What can Janice do to help her colleagues "unfreeze" and give more serious consideration to strengthening the leadership focus throughout the curriculum?
2. What leader characteristics would be most beneficial to Janice as she strives to strengthen the curriculum in ways that will help graduates take responsibility for being leaders themselves?

that eliminates specialty silos, focuses on integration, is open and flexible, attends more to competency than to "seat time," and engages teachers and students as co-learners, faculty colleagues may need extended time to prepare for and implement such a change. The leader might circulate articles or books that address the need to transform nursing education (and health professions education in general), negotiate with administrators to bring experts to the school to talk about their experiences with creating and implementing such curricula, provide extensive opportunities for dialogue and expression of concern about the change, and outline a clear timeline of the steps that need to be taken to achieve the goal in a reasonable time frame.

In contrast to evolutionary change processes, faculty who are early adopters of various technologies and appreciate the need to fully integrate technology into the educational program may promote a more revolutionary approach to change. They may gather together to form a group to pilot various teaching/learning technologies, document the outcomes of those "experiments," make revisions based on the outcomes, report findings to the larger faculty, encourage and mentor others to try new approaches in their courses, and continue to move ahead with integrating the technology even if everyone else is not "on board."

Whichever approach to change is used, the leader must take the risk of offering new ideas or approaches, influencing others to "get on board," and collaborating with followers to sustain the change. This influence is needed within the school/program, but it is needed on a broad level as well.

PARTICIPATE IN INTERDISCIPLINARY EFFORTS; ADAPT TO CHANGES CREATED BY EXTERNAL FACTORS; CREATE A CULTURE FOR CHANGE

Effective nursing education leaders have a broad perspective, are not limited in their thinking, are aware of external forces that impact nursing education, learn from colleagues in other fields, and work to create a preferred future within their own program, the larger institution, the community, and the field in general. They serve on institutional committees that address educational standards, outcomes assessment, educational innovations, student engagement, or ongoing development of the pedagogical expertise of faculty. They read the educational literature and follow education-focused listserv/discussion groups while keeping current in the clinical areas that they teach. They attend conferences related to nursing and health professions education, curriculum development, program evaluation, educational technology, and issues in higher education, and they participate in national organizations that focus on shaping nursing and higher education.

Nursing education leaders also initiate discussions of appointment, promotion, and tenure criteria to heighten awareness of the need to recognize and reward excellence and innovation in teaching, leadership in curriculum development, and the scholarship of teaching and learning—not only the traditional activities of research, grant funding, and peer-reviewed publications. Such discussions can take place within one's school or institution or at regional and national levels. Does action such as this involve risk? Indeed, it does. However, as noted earlier, leaders are risk takers who often say what needs to be said and challenge traditional ways of thinking and the status quo.

In addition to these activities, nursing education leaders are involved politically. They advocate for funding to support educational innovations, faculty development, and pedagogical research. They meet with legislators in the local community, at the state level, or at the national level to educate political figures about the nature of our work as educators, the focus of nursing education, the significance and challenges of clinical learning experiences, and the need for evidence-based teaching practices, among other issues. Some also may assume roles as political leaders to ensure that they are "at the table" and in a position to bring the wisdom, insights, and perspectives of nurse educators to significant issues under discussion.

Finally, it is important that nursing education leaders serve as mentors to others desiring to shape a preferred future for the field. Providing opportunities for faculty colleagues to co-lead change efforts; experiment with new approaches to teaching/learning; or develop proposals for a new committee structure, advisement system, or revised curriculum are ways that a leader can mentor others. The leader also can encourage colleagues who share the passion for educational innovation to become involved in organizations that shape the field at the national level. Additionally, the leader can mentor other faculty by inviting them to co-author publications or co-present papers at conferences.

Scenario 6.3

Luciana is a full professor on the clinical track in a research-intensive institution who teaches, advises students, serves on committees, and is engaged in scholarly work related to nursing education. She has received several grants to support pedagogical research studies; published in education-focused, peer-reviewed journals; presented at national and international conferences; is actively involved in professional organizations that advance excellence in nursing education; provides consultation to schools of nursing on teaching/learning, faculty development, and other education topics; and has received awards and Academy inductions in recognition of her sustained contributions to and leadership in nursing education. Luciana wants to help other faculty develop as education scholars who engage in *scholarly teaching* by basing their teaching practices on evidence and who engage in the *scholarship of teaching* to advance the science of nursing education. She decides to schedule several informal discussion sessions, invite faculty who desire to grow as education scholars, and "get the ball rolling" to propose ways in which the school of nursing can build its capacity for pedagogical research to complement the level of excellence that it has achieved related to clinical research.

Consider:
1. What risks is Luciana taking as she proposes these ideas?
2. What kind of support and mentoring will junior faculty need to be part of this initiative and develop as education scholars?
3. What can Luciana do to see that such support is provided?
4. How can she use her professional networks within the school, university, and profession to help advance this faculty development effort?

SUMMARY

It should be clear from this discussion that nursing education leaders look outward, not inward. They envision new ways to approach nursing education, implement the faculty role, or engage students actively in the learning process. They express this vision clearly and with passion. They work with followers—individuals who also support the vision—and with key stakeholders (e.g., students, clinical partners, faculty from other disciplines, administrators, legislators) to design and implement the changes needed to realize the vision. They feel a sense of accomplishment when excellence is defined and achieved.

Every faculty member needs to think of themselves as a leader and not abdicate that responsibility to the dean, program director, or department chairperson. Nursing faculty are role models for students and prepare students to be leaders in nursing. Therefore, they must be willing to take the risk of being leaders themselves, individuals who envision a preferred future, articulate that vision with passion, engage and empower others to help achieve the vision, facilitate change that will benefit students and colleagues as well as nursing education itself, and live a commitment to excellence.

Practice Test Questions

1. Which explanation highlights the differences between leaders and managers?
   A. Leaders focus on task accomplishment; managers focus on long-term goals.
   B. Leaders' power comes from their role in the organization; managers' power comes from their knowledge.
   C. Leaders' goals arise from a passion for excellence; managers' goals arise from those of the organization.
   D. Leaders direct subordinates in their work; managers collaborate with followers.

2. What action is best for the nurse educator leader to effectively role model cultural sensitivity when advocating for change?
   A. Invite all members of the faculty to respond to a survey about the need for the change.
   B. Acknowledge that the background and unique perspectives of each member influence how each will react to a proposed change.
   C. Ask representatives from various faculty subgroups (e.g., tenured/nontenured, educated in/outside the United States) to review a proposed change prior to presenting it to the full faculty.
   D. Attend lectures about diversity and cultural differences.

3. Which action would be most effective in helping the nursing education leader evaluate the readiness of colleagues for transformative change in the curriculum?
   A. Review the evaluations completed by faculty who attended a presentation on curriculum development.
   B. Determine the nature and extent of change experienced by the group in recent years and the support provided by administration for the change.
   C. Reflect on the extent to which comments made at a meeting are congruent with one's own goals.
   D. Interview faculty regarding their nursing practice experiences.

4. The nurse educator reflects on recent higher education literature about empowering students and envisions a prelicensure program that gives students some choice regarding the assignments that they complete for a course and the percentage each will count toward the course grade. By doing this, what is the nurse educator helping to shape?
   A. New workload calculation practices
   B. Collaborative relationships with clinical partners
   C. A preferred future for nursing education
   D. Standards for program evaluation

5. Based on characteristics that describe effective leaders, which action will the nurse educator use to facilitate change and innovation?
   A. Clearly articulate a vision and motivate others to help realize that vision.
   B. Achieve tenure and seek a position of authority in an organization.
   C. Chair an important committee in the school and hold the rank of professor.
   D. Provide clear directions to others in completing tasks and set a prescribed timeline for implementation.

6. Effective followers display which set of characteristics?
   A. Keep focused on the present; ensure that policies are implemented as prescribed.
   B. Challenge new ideas; support members of the group who advocate maintaining the status quo.
   C. Accept tasks assigned by the leader without question; listen to all discussions about the new initiative.
   D. Collaborate with the leader to design activities to meet the goal; think critically.

7. Which responsibility may be assumed by the nurse leader who is *not* in a formal position of authority (i.e., dean, chair, etc.) in the school?
   A. Lead strategic planning efforts for the school as a whole
   B. Develop and oversee implementation of the school's budget
   C. Help members of the faculty engage in evidence-based teaching practices
   D. Serve as the spokesperson for the school within the parent institution

8. Which action by the nurse educator best demonstrates the role of leader and change agent?
   A. Accept an invitation to run for office in a national organization.
   B. Continue to work in the ICU at least one weekend per month.
   C. Advocate to retain the curriculum plan, citing no major negative outcomes of it.
   D. Inform students of the benefits of scholarly work.

9. Which action by the nurse educator would best demonstrate leadership and enhance the visibility of nursing in the parent institution?
   A. Serve as chair of the school's student affairs committee.
   B. Volunteer at a local indigent care clinic.
   C. Attend the institution's faculty senate meetings.
   D. Coordinate a health fair for faculty and staff of the parent institution.

10. First-time pass rates on the licensing exam at the school have been below the national average for the past two years. The newly appointed chair believes that curriculum revision is necessary to address this situation. Drawing on knowledge of Lewin's change theory, what is the most likely problem that the new chair will encounter in beginning to advocate for curriculum change?
   A. Policies that prevent new approaches during the data-gathering stage
   B. Resistance during the unfreezing stage
   C. Sabotage during the refreezing stage
   D. Lack of financial support during the moving stage

References

Christensen, C. M., Raynor, M., & McDonald, R. (2015). What is disruptive innovation? *Harvard Business Review, 93*(12), 44–53.

Clark, C. (2017). *Creating & sustaining civility in nursing education* (2nd ed.). Indianapolis, IN: Sigma Theta Tau International Honor Society of Nursing.

Grossman, S. C., & Valiga, T. M. (2017). *The new leadership challenge: Creating the future of nursing* (5th ed.). Philadelphia, PA: F. A. Davis.

Lewin, K. (1951). *Field theory in social science: Selected theoretical papers.* New York, NY: Harper & Row.

National League for Nursing Certification Commission Certification Test Development Committee. (2012). *The scope of practice for academic nurse educators* (2012 revision). New York, NY: National League for Nursing.

Zaleznik, A. (1981). Managers and leaders: Are they different? *Journal of Nursing Administration, 11*(7), 25–31.

7

Engage in Scholarship of Teaching

Marilyn Frenn, PhD, RN, CNE, FTOS, ANEF, FAAN

The CNE Test Plan lists the following for the area of Engage in Scholarship of Teaching:

B. Engage in Scholarship of Teaching
1. Exhibit a spirit of inquiry about teaching and learning, student development, and evaluation methods.
2. Use evidence-based resources to improve and support teaching.
3. Participate in research activities related to nursing education.
4. Share teaching expertise with colleagues and others.
5. Demonstrate integrity as a scholar.

The activities noted in the detailed CNE® test blueprint for Category 6B reflect the nurse educator's role related to the scholarship of teaching. As noted, there are five major areas covered in this section, each equally important to the scholarship of teaching.

EXHIBIT A SPIRIT OF INQUIRY ABOUT TEACHING AND LEARNING, STUDENT DEVELOPMENT, AND EVALUATION METHODS

A spirit of inquiry is within the nature of a scholar. A scholar is a member of a profession who is able to think logically and is a self-directed thinker. The scholar is able to develop new ideas and approaches in an attempt to solve problems of the profession. An important element of a scholar is engaging in lifelong learning about an area of expertise. Although knowledgeable about all areas of nursing education, any single faculty member cannot be an expert in all. Therefore, a scholar identifies an area of personal interest and engages in scholarly activities related to that interest. We collectively advance the science through rigorous inquiry (Patterson et al., 2018), as shown in Box 7.1.

In his classic work, Boyer (1990) describes four dimensions of scholarship that provide an important foundation for understanding perspectives on the nature of inquiry. Boyer described discovery, integration, application, and teaching as dimensions of scholarship in higher education.

Discovery is associated with epistemologies most commonly known as research. Boyer (1990) described this dimension of inquiry as "demonstrating palpable excitement in the life of the institution" (p. 17).

- The National League for Nursing (NLN, 2019b) has funded nursing education research for almost two decades, sets research priorities (2016), and has sponsored a center for the advancement of the science of nursing education since 2012.

BOX 7.1 Scholarly Attributes of the Academic Nurse Educator
The academic nurse educator (Patterson & McLaughlin, 2019): • Draws on extant literature to design evidence-based teaching and evaluation practices • Exhibits a spirit of inquiry about teaching and learning, student development, evaluation methods, and other aspects of the role • Designs and implements scholarly activities in an established area of expertise • Disseminates nursing and teaching knowledge to a variety of audiences through various means • Demonstrates skill in proposal writing for initiatives that include—but are not limited to—research, resource acquisition, program development, and policy development • Demonstrates qualities of a scholar—integrity, courage, perseverance, vitality, and creativity

- The competencies underlying the Certified Nurse Educator (CNE®) examination are evidence based (Halstead, 2019) and have been used to guide research (Frenn & Dreifuerst, 2019).
- Similarly, the World Health Organization (2016, p. 13) developed competencies based on a Delphi survey. The fourth of 13 competencies states, "Nurse educators develop their critical inquiry and the ability to conduct research and utilize findings to identify and solve educational and practice-based problems."
- Nurse educators may begin with pilot studies (Spurlock, 2018b), building larger multisite studies with adequate statistical power as warranted to advance the science (Taylor & Spurlock, 2018) beyond single-group pretest–posttest designs that have limited utility in testing interventions (Spurlock, 2018a).

The scholarship of integration is a process of pulling together isolated facts in a meaningful way to generate new insights. Building bridges across disciplinary knowledge is an example that Boyer (1990) gave in which insights might be generated in this dimension. The notion of scholarship incorporates the idea that the work is judged as meritorious by worthy peers.

- Nurse educators need a solid foundation in nursing knowledge as well as theories of learning and of the disciplines that intersect in order to further develop and integrate that knowledge into teaching (Beccaria, Kek, & Huijser, 2018).
- Systematic reviews and meta-analyses or meta-syntheses are useful to evaluate and integrate knowledge beyond a single study. For example, both concept mapping (Yue, Zhang, Zhang, & Jin, 2017) and an evidence-based nursing approach (Cui, Li, Geng, Zhang, & Jin, 2018) were found to increase students' critical thinking in meta-analyses.
- Scholarly teaching requires critical reflection and integration of published research into curricula and course content, as well as mentoring of students (Bullin, 2018).

The scholarship of application is putting knowledge to use in addressing consequential problems (Boyer, 1990). Rather than doing social good or being a good citizen, *per se*, scholarship of application requires action flowing from faculty members' expertise. The action, in turn, informs their body of knowledge and accumulated expertise.

- Though laudable, service that is unrelated to teaching expertise would not be scholarship of application.

- Clinical scholarship wherein knowledge produced is peer reviewed, documented, and disseminated could be scholarship of application (Limoges & Acorn, 2016). Examples include development of guidelines and policy papers related to practice.
- Teaching itself is the final dimension of scholarship (Boyer, 1990), flowing from Aristotle's view that teaching is the highest form of understanding. Scholarly teaching transforms knowledge, extending it through students who are critical and creative thinkers long after the learning has occurred.
- Teaching can be turned into scholarship by reflecting on teaching, searching the literature, planning improvements, evaluating, and publishing and/or other means of dissemination based on the improvements (Oermann, 2017).
- Scholarship of teaching and learning (SoTL) can also be used in curriculum revision (Landeen et al., 2016; Nosek, Scheckel, Waterbury, Macdonald, & Wozney, 2017). Review of the literature for curriculum change, incorporation of pertinent theories, implementation, evaluation using rigorous research methods, and dissemination comprise this approach.

Colleagues in other disciplines also provided examples that could be used by nurse educators:

- A professional writing course that could be used by others (Miller, Grise-Owens, Drury, & Rickman, 2018)
- An interdisciplinary learning community incorporating service learning and other theoretically based active learning approaches (Weaver, Haak, Molt, & Cannon, 2018).

Beyond having a spirit of inquiry only about teaching and learning, the CNE examination blueprint, based on the Nurse Educator Competencies (Halstead, 2019) indicates that nursing education scholarship also focuses on student development and evaluation methods, both of which are covered in other sections of this book.

- Nursing education scholarship increasingly needs to address student development and evaluation related to interprofessional education (IPE). The Institute of Medicine (2010) report on the future of nursing called for IPE wherein students from different disciplines learn together. The Interprofessional Education Collaborative (2016) released core competencies, including role/responsibility development, interprofessional communication, and team building to improve client outcomes.
- The NLN (2016) nursing education research priorities incorporate requisites for IPE as well as nursing-specific educational inquiry. The NLN also published a book to facilitate incorporation of IPE in nursing education (Speakman, 2016).

Scenario 7.1

Following pilot work in her own school trying an educational innovation, the nurse educator worked with a team to test the innovation across several schools using instruments with acceptable estimates of reliability and validity and a sufficient sample, as determined by power analysis. This is an example of which of Boyer's dimensions of scholarship?

Consider: This is an example of the scholarship of discovery!

USE EVIDENCE-BASED RESOURCES TO IMPROVE AND SUPPORT TEACHING

The second aspect to be reviewed in preparation for the CNE examination relates to use of evidence-based resources to improve and support teaching. The complexities of the work that students are prepared for and the science undergirding our understanding of learning demand that educators move beyond the pedagogies within which they were taught to use evidence-based teaching strategies (Culyer, Jatulis, Cannistraci, & Brownell, 2018).

- Evidence-based teaching (EBT) is defined as "a dynamic, holistic system using educational principles validated by evidence to support, maintain, and promote a new level of knowledge for a learner in a variety of settings" (Boswell & Cannon, 2016).
- Beyond the evidence base, *per se*, it is important to consider the nurse educator's experience and student learning needs in applying the evidence (Oermann, 2018).
- An example is to use cognitive rehearsal through simulation to better prepare students to address patient safety issues in a way that fosters respectful communication in the workplace (Clark, 2019). Specific theory and evidence guide each step of preparing students, developing or obtaining a simulation script, prebriefing, and debriefing.
- Oermann (2018) noted that we have evidence on flipped classrooms and other active learning approaches, as well as systematic reviews and meta-analyses on simulation. She cited the need for more research on clinical nursing and interprofessional clinical education both across institutions and within one's own clinical course.
- In reviewing the evidence for use of the NLN Core Competencies of Nurse Educators, studies using instruments with acceptable estimates of reliability and validity were found. However, investigators did not use those instruments consistently, and those applying findings in practice often developed their own surveys to examine outcomes rather than use the available instruments (Frenn & Dreifuerst, 2019).
- Studies often lacked rigor, had small sample sizes, and had not been replicated across settings. Although there were many qualitative and descriptive studies, researchers had not defined concepts or operationalized them in the same manner across studies. Randomized controlled studies with sufficient statistical power comparing educational interventions are needed (Frenn & Dreifuerst, 2019).
- Better funding for nursing education research along with nursing research is much needed.
- Meanwhile, collaborative studies across educational institutions, replication using the same instruments, and dissemination of curricular evaluation findings could help. Oermann (2017) pointed out that the evidence should first be consulted as innovations are developed, evaluation should be planned from the start, and results disseminated.
- The conduct and dissemination of rigorous systematic reviews using established criteria (e.g., as proposed by Im & Chang, 2012; Morin, 2012; and Whittemore & Knafl, 2005) may make evidence more available for use.
- Barriers to EBT were lack of time and administrative and peer support, as well as large classes (Culyer et al., 2018). Similar to the factors that Melnyk, Fineout-Overholt, Gallagher-Ford, and Kaplan (2012) noted that improved evidence-based practice (EBP), an organizational culture that empowered faculty fostered EBT.

- Similar to EBP, frameworks have been proposed for evidence-based nursing education. Emerson and Records (2008) proposed the Student, Teaching technique, Comparison, and Outcome format. Boswell and Cannon (2016) reviewed models of EBP and proposed a format for evidence-based nursing education, including Population (students, administrators, faculty, alumni, candidates, preceptors, or others), Strategy, Comparison, Outcome, and Time period when applicable.
- A first step when appraising research for evidence-based nursing education is clearly stating the question: What teaching/learning practice, curricular innovation, or student development issue requires evidence for decision-making? Databases such as the Cumulative Index for Nursing and Allied Health (CINAHL), Dissertation Abstracts, PubMed, PsychINFO, Educational Resources Information Center (ERIC), and Cochrane—along with the help of a skilled reference librarian—are essential for locating studies. Careful decision-making is needed about years to include, search words, and the quality of studies or other manuscripts. Search the reference lists for additional relevant studies and use the database functions to examine articles citing the most useful studies and studies similar to them. Often, authors use different terminology than a researcher may use when conducting a search; thus, finding one relevant study can lead to others.
- An evidence table is helpful for organizing results of a literature search. See Table 7.1 for an example nursing education evidence table. In the table, it is important to note the following: research question, the databases searched, the citations, subjects (type of students, demographics), method, results, whether the study was applicable (to the setting, students, faculty, other stakeholders, congruent with laws, accreditation standards, organizational mission, and ethical standards), your rating of the quality of the evidence in that study, and any information on the cost to implement the findings in the educational setting. The bottom of the table provides a space to state recommendations based on all of the studies and to rate the quality of the overall evidence leading to the recommendation. If there are many studies, a better approach may be to prepare a final table with only the studies of good quality that are pertinent and applicable.

Table 7.1

Evidence-Based Nursing Education Appraisal

What is your specific teaching/learning, curriculum, student progress question?

What key words, databases, years will be searched?

Citation	Subjects	Method	Measures	Results	Applicable	Strength of Evidence	Cost?

Recommendation:

Strength of <u>overall</u> evidence:

BOX 7.2   Elements for Consideration in Appraising Qualitative Nursing Education Research

- Is the design appropriate for the research question(s)?
- Was a thorough, in-depth, intensive examination of the study aims conducted?
- Were the rights of study participants protected, including review by an institutional review board?
- Did the sample provide rich data with sufficient time spent to yield saturation of categories?
- Was the qualitative method consistently and rigorously applied with sufficient reflexivity to prevent bias?
- Do the themes appear to parsimoniously capture the meaning of the narratives?
- Does the report give you a clear and meaningful picture of the world of study participants?

- A tool to evaluate integrative reviews (Health Evidence, 2013) can be used to examine EBT. Example integrative reviews include those related to Universal Design for Instruction (Levey, 2018), flipped classrooms (Njie-Carr et al., 2017), and preparing students for the emotional challenges of nursing (Dwyer & Revell, 2015).
- When appraising individual nursing education studies, research texts (e.g., Polit & Beck, 2017) can be consulted. See Boxes 7.2 and 7.3 for a quick

---

BOX 7.3   Elements for Consideration in Appraising Quantitative Nursing Education Research

- Were the sample size and selection criteria sufficient for statistical power?
- Was the strongest design used as appropriate for the research question?
- Was a clearly identified conceptual framework used to guide choice of variables and educational interventions?
- Were reliability and validity estimates for instruments provided and acceptable?
- Were the rights of study participants protected, including review by an institutional review board?
- Was fidelity to the intervention (if applicable) assured and diffusion to the control prevented?
- Was the timing of the collection of data appropriate?
- Was adequate masking/blinding used for intervention and control groups?
- Were statistics used appropriate for the level of measurement: that is, nominal, ordinal, interval, or ratio levels?
- Were conclusions supported by the data?

Scenario 7.2

To engage their educational community in evidence-based teaching, a group of nurse educators develop the following (Boswell & Cannon, 2016):

P (Population): Prelicensure students
S (Strategy): Planned evaluation based on objectives
C (Comparisons): Pop quizzes
O (Outcome): Student test scores
T (Time Period): None used

After reviewing the evidence, the nurse educators found that pop quizzes were an ineffective approach.

Consider: What evaluation characteristics are important to consider? Effective evaluation is planned from the start, and students are told when and how their learning will be evaluated.

review of elements to consider when appraising qualitative and quantitative nursing education research. The Joanna Briggs Institute (http://joannabriggs.org/) also provides a process and electronic tools for appraisal and synthesis of health-related evidence.

- Recent studies provide helpful examples of the application of evidence in nursing education. Nurse educators and administrators ($N = 551$) reported that EBT was important to address student learning needs and build the science of nursing education (Kalb, O'Conner-Von, Brockway, Rierson, & Sendelbach, 2015). Simulation is an evidence-based teaching approach, but nurse educators' self-efficacy is important in using it to improve student outcomes (Garner et al., 2018).

PARTICIPATE IN RESEARCH ACTIVITIES RELATED TO NURSING EDUCATION

The third aspect of scholarship of teaching examined in the CNE examination is participation in research activities. Besides conducting individual or collaborative nursing education studies, faculty members can contribute by raising questions about current practices. See Box 7.4 for additional ideas. Further testing with valid and reliable instruments is needed.

- Oermann (2009) noted that many educational practices are untested. Questions can be used to formulate the basis for a literature search, systematic review, or conversation among colleagues that may catalyze development of a symposium or conference session bringing together those with the greatest expertise on the topic of concern. An article about a useful practice can be written (Van Der Like, Fox, Blackburn, & Chisholm, 2019). Questions may also inform evaluations of current practices.

BOX 7.4 Participating in Research Activities Related to Nursing Education

Formal processes can be created to stimulate attention to nursing education research.

- Nurse educators can create a research brief component to faculty meetings, talking about the meaning of the findings for nursing education (Spurlock Jr., 2017).
- Faculty can take turns reporting on relevant research for their curriculum or student issues, or issues in higher education.
- When admission and progression policies are discussed, a taskforce can be created to examine relevant studies. Faculty teaching in similar areas can send new study citations and abstracts of interest by email, putting application questions on a future meeting agenda.
- Senior faculty and administrators can advocate that evidence-based teaching is a component of promotion and tenure requirements. They can mentor others in evidence-based teaching.
- All faculty members can share interesting studies by mentioning them to colleagues, leaving a copy on the lunchroom table or other common areas.
- Nursing education research requires much more funding to support larger, multisite studies. Faculty can inform funding agencies and policy makers of this need to ensure quality nursing education.
- They can also contribute to and commend organizations funding nursing education research. The NLN, Sigma Theta Tau International, and the Midwest Nursing Research Society are a few of the organizations funding dissertation and other nursing education research.

- Evaluations require a valid and reliable instrument(s) (Spurlock, 2017). Faculty can participate in instrument development studies to develop tools for later use. They may participate as subjects (Raymond, Profetto-McGrath, Myrick, & Strean, 2018) or as content experts, contributing to face or content validity indices. Since grades could be used in program, course, or educational innovation evaluation, faculty can advocate for equal interval grade scales. Often, grading scales are developed without rationale, and a more useful purpose can be made of the data generated every semester. When nonequal intervals are used, ordinal-level statistics must be used to analyze the data. These statistics are not as commonly used, and the power to predict statistically significant results is diminished compared with interval-level statistics (Polit & Beck, 2017).

- In 2003, the NLN Task Group on Teaching Learning proposed many ways that faculty members can help to build the science of nursing education. Central to these approaches are a questioning spirit and critical mind. Developing frameworks for the practice of teaching, databases to organize evidence, and measurable outcomes of nursing education are examples provided by Gresley (2009). Faculty members may also demonstrate skill in proposal writing for initiatives such as research, resources, and program and policy development to build the science of nursing education (Halstead, 2007). Or faculty may engage students using social media, such as Twitter (Stephens & Gunther, 2016).

Scenario 7.3

Stephen joined the faculty at a small liberal arts college where conduct of research is not part of his workload. To help build the science of nursing education, he contributes to foundations that support nursing education research and participates in studies to develop new instruments to evaluate educational innovations.

Consider: Which of Boyer's dimensions of scholarship is Stephen addressing? The scholarship of application is exemplified by meaningful service related to the nurse educator's area of expertise; thus, Stephen is demonstrating the scholarship of application.

SHARE TEACHING EXPERTISE WITH COLLEAGUES AND OTHERS

The fourth component of Scholarship of Teaching on the CNE examination is sharing teaching expertise with colleagues and others. Skilled teachers incorporate evidence-based nursing education seamlessly. They discern which aspects of the evidence are critical to student success in their program, preparing them for lifelong learning and effective practice. Sharing this wisdom with a variety of audiences constitutes this aspect of engaging in nursing education scholarship (Halstead, 2007).

- Expertise can be shared in various ways throughout a nursing education career (Halstead, 2007). Novice educators may engage in course work to better understand teaching, learning, and curricular initiatives. They bring fresh perspectives to discussions with colleagues about the application of pedagogical theories and research to the preparation of nurses for current practice. Novice educators may try out approaches based in the literature, discussing options and outcomes with colleagues. More experienced educators may mentor novice faculty, sharing their emerging synthesis of evidence-based nursing education along with clinical, institutional, and financial realities. Teaching expertise may be recognized through certification as a nurse educator, awards, endowed chairs, and special appointments as the faculty member develops (Adams & Valiga, 2009).

- Pedagogical expertise should be developed in all doctoral programs (Booth, Emerson, Hackney, & Souter, 2016). Teaching expertise was positively correlated with nurse educators' intent to stay in the academic organization (Candela, Gutierrez, & Keating, 2015).
- The highest-impact initiatives may involve actualizing teaching expertise in program development and institutional initiatives, such as service learning (VanGraafeiland, Sloand, Silbert-Flagg, Gleason, & Dennison Himmelfarb, 2019), first-year seminars, and capstone projects (Hutchings, Huber, & Ciccone, 2011). With this approach, faculty learn from reflecting on how their efforts have worked to improve student outcomes, then share this information with interdisciplinary colleagues, thereby further developing knowledge.

Scenario 7.4

Sharon has been teaching N2000 Introduction to Clinical Nursing for five years, integrating the literature each time she taught the course. She is now asked to mentor a new nurse educator who will be teaching a section of the course. Sharon acknowledges that peer mentoring has been found to be effective and makes a series of appointments with her new colleague to share aspects of the course that have worked well and suggestions she is using for improvement, as well as to talk about developing in the faculty role. She shares her approach to evaluating students and offers to talk with her colleague as students work to meet clinical objectives.

Consider: Sharon is engaged in which of Boyer's dimensions of scholarship? The scholarship of integration entails pulling together knowledge in ways that generate new insights; thus, the scholarship of integration is most closely exemplified by what Sharon is sharing with her colleague.

DEMONSTRATE INTEGRITY AS A SCHOLAR

While performing all of the aspects of engaging in the scholarship of teaching, demonstrating integrity is essential. Engaging in the scholarship of teaching means that faculty understand what is known, examine it, and discover and create new ways of knowing. The more faculty understand, the greater the obligation as scholars to use this knowledge and skill with the integration of "mind and moral virtue" that is called integrity (Shulman, 2008, p. ix). As a component of the NLN's (2019a) core values, integrity is defined as "respecting the dignity and moral wholeness of every person without conditions or limitation." Integrity has also been described as the congruence between what we say and how we act (Simons, 1999). For example, when teaching cultural competence, it is important that nurse educators do their best to involve students with culturally diverse teams (Rozelle, 2018) and communities (Alexander-Ruff & Kinion, 2019).

- Theories of ethics provide us with guidance for action (Bosek & Savage, 2007). Many institutions of higher learning follow the American Association of University Professors (2009) Statement on Professional Ethics (Smith, 2012). This statement includes engaging in intellectual honesty, being a role model of ethical standards, protecting students' academic freedom, maintaining confidentiality and refraining from exploitation or discriminatory behaviors, respecting the inquiry of associates, demonstrating collegiality and responsibility for institutional governance, discriminating between action as an individual and institutional representative, and being effective teachers and scholars. Fostering cultural competency is important in nursing education scholarship and in being effective teachers and scholars (Wesp et al., 2018). Best practice requires that faculty socialize students to professional ethical standards (Smith, 2012), which means that nursing faculty incorporate ethics as both nurse and faculty member (Cannon & Boswell, 2016).

- Though some nonresearch educational inquiries may not require ratification by an institutional review board, because of the power that faculty members have over students, it is wise to have the protocol reviewed for the protection of students (Aycock & Currie, 2013; Kragelund, 2013). As a vulnerable population, students must be able to choose to participate or be able to decline participation as research subjects with reasonable alternatives available to them. Engaging a research assistant not involved with the course to collect consent documents and hold them until the course is finished can provide additional assurance that students are able to freely ask questions.

- Involving students as subjects or as co-investigators, or mentoring them in their own research studies, contributes greatly to the evolution of nursing education science and development of the skills of scholarship. Modeling integrity and ethical comportment (American Nurses Association, 2015) in the work of faculty provides a more effective message than any content or value taught. It is so exciting to have former students encounter you at professional meetings letting you know that they are pursuing further education as a result of the time spent with you.

Scenario 7.5

A student tells the nurse educator that she is unwilling to share information about various treatment options with a client because some of the options are incongruent with the student's religious beliefs.

Consider: How might the nurse educator demonstrate integrity as a scholar in addressing this? At a clinical conference, the nurse educator could raise the issue, asking students to pull from the literature professional codes of ethics and state board requirements regarding care that may conflict with personal beliefs. The opportunity for other students to engage in the patient teaching could then be discussed with the client's nurse so that that the learning opportunity could be given to another student willing and prepared to discuss treatment options with the client.

SUMMARY

Resources for the NLN Nurse Educator Competency "Engage in Scholarship of Teaching" have been reviewed in this chapter. Each of the following aspects are equally important to prepare the next generation of nurses: exhibit a spirit of inquiry; use evidence-based resources to improve and support teaching; participate in nursing education research activities; share teaching expertise; and demonstrate integrity as a scholar. Help create the future of nursing!

Practice Test Questions

1. Which action best demonstrates the scholarship of discovery?
   A. Conducts an original research study that results in the identification of new knowledge.
   B. Designs learning models that facilitate learner application of previous knowledge.
   C. Uses a variety of teaching methods to actively engage learners.
   D. Applies evidence in service as an organizational leader.

2. Based on Boyer's Model of Scholarship, which faculty activity fulfills a scholarship of discovery?
   A. Develop a criterion-referenced examination using items written at the application and analysis level of Bloom's taxonomy.
   B. Share at a state conference expertise on the application of genetics in nursing.
   C. Evaluate a novice in the nursing college using a self-developed rubric based on educational research.
   D. Examine the effectiveness of problem-based team case studies in achieving positive learning outcomes in a multisite study.

3. A new faculty member would like to better engage in the scholarship of teaching. Which is the best action to initiate?
   A. Run for a faculty senator position.
   B. Organize an ethnocentric learning experience.
   C. Present the outcomes of a service-learning project.
   D. Practice as a registered nurse one weekend a month.

4. A nurse educator has accepted an appointment as a Strategic Steering Committee member at the National League for Nursing. Which scholarship role is the nursing educator fulfilling?
   A. Application
   B. Integration
   C. Discovery
   D. Teaching

5. Which activity would a nurse educator use in a portfolio to demonstrate the Scholarship of Application?
   A. Evaluations of the work by colleagues that was published in a refereed journal
   B. Any type of service, such as volunteering at the animal shelter every week all year
   C. Reporting on a health fair for the community so that students could interact with people
   D. Description of how the work broadened the professor's understanding of the field

6. Which would provide the best example of evidence-based teaching?
   A. Developing an educational innovation based on one's own BSN student experience
   B. Conducting a literature review using established criteria
   C. Teaching the course as it always has been taught
   D. Teaching the course without regard to student perspectives

7. What would best demonstrate sharing of teaching expertise?
   A. Course syllabi for the past seven years
   B. Educational programs the educator has attended
   C. Transcripts demonstrating course work related to nursing education
   D. The educator's publications related to evaluated teaching innovations

8. A student stated the intention not to inform a patient about aspects of health care that were incongruent with the student's religious beliefs. The nurse educator provides feedback to the student that client autonomy must be respected. What best describes this feedback?
   A. This demonstrates integrity as a scholar, since protecting client autonomy is included in professional nursing ethics.
   B. The nurse educator violated the student's rights to free speech by providing this feedback.
   C. The faculty member should insist that the student change the religious belief or be removed from the program.
   D. Client autonomy must be respected only if the client is being asked to participate in research.

9. The nurse educator wants to include current students in a study the educator is planning to conduct. Which statement about education research bears on this situation?
   A. Since this is part of the faculty role, no review for protection of human subjects is required.
   B. The nurse educator must pay students involved in research.
   C. The nurse educator hires a research assistant who collects consent documents approved by the institutional review board and does not see the deidentified data until the semester has ended.
   D. Since the information collected is so important, all students are informed that they must participate.

10. What has the National League for Nursing done to foster development of nursing education science?
    A. Fund nursing education research
    B. Establish priorities for nursing education research
    C. A and B
    D. Neither A nor B

References

Adams, M. H., & Valiga, T. M. (Eds.). (2009). *Achieving excellence in nursing education*. New York, NY: National League for Nursing.

Alexander-Ruff, J. H., & Kinion, E. S. (2019). Developing a cultural immersion service-learning experience for undergraduate nursing students. *Journal of Nursing Education, 58*(2), 117–120. doi:10.3928/01484834-20190122-11

American Association of University Professors. (2009). Statement on professional ethics. Retrieved from http://www.aaup.org/report/statement-professional-ethics

American Nurses Association. (2015). Code of ethics with interpretative statements. Retrieved from: https://www.nursingworld.org/practice-policy/nursing-excellence/ethics/code-of-ethics-for-nurses/

Aycock, D. M., & Currie, E. R. (2013). Minimizing risks for nursing students recruited for health and educational research. *Nurse Educator, 38*(2), 56–60. doi: 10.1097/NNE.0b013e3182829c3a

Beccaria, L., Kek, M. Y. C. A., & Huijser, H. (2018). Exploring nursing educators' use of theory and methods in search for evidence based credibility in nursing education. *Nurse Education Today, 65*, 60–66. doi:10.1016/j.nedt.2018.02.032

Booth, T. L., Emerson, C. J., Hackney, M. G., & Souter, S. (2016). Preparation of academic nurse educators. *Nurse Education in Practice, 19*, 54–57. doi:10.1016/j.nepr.2016.04.006

Bosek, M. S. D., & Savage, T. A. (2007). *The ethical component of nursing education*. Philadelphia, PA: Lippincott Williams & Wilkins.

Boswell, C., & Cannon, S. (2016). Overview of evidence-based practice. In S. Cannon & C. Boswell (Eds.), *Evidence-based teaching in nursing: A foundation for educators* (2nd ed.). Burlington, MA: Jones & Bartlett Learning.

Boyer, E. (1990). *Scholarship reconsidered: Priorities for the professoriate*. Princeton, NJ: The Carnegie Foundation for the Advancement of Teaching.

Brown, R., Taylor, M. J., & Geddes, J. (2013). Aripiprazole alone or in combination for acute mania. *Cochrane Database of Systematic Reviews*, (12). doi:10.1002/14651858. CD005000.pub2. (Accession No. CD005000)

Bullin, C. (2018). To what extent has doctoral (PhD) education supported academic nurse educators in their teaching roles: An integrative review. *BMC Nursing, 17*, 1–18. doi:10.1186/s12912-018-0273-3

Candela, L., Gutierrez, A. P., & Keating, S. (2015). What predicts nurse faculty members' intent to stay in the academic organization? A structural equation model of a national survey of nursing faculty. *Nurse Education Today, 35*(4), 580–589. doi:10.1016/j.nedt.2014.12.018

Cannon, S., & Boswell, C. (Eds.). (2016). *Evidence-based teaching in nursing: A foundation for educators* (2nd ed.). Burlington, MA: Jones & Bartlett.

Clark, C. M. (2019). Combining cognitive rehearsal, simulation, and evidence-based scripting to address incivility. *Nurse Educator, 44*(2), 64–68. doi:10.1097/NNE.0000000000000563

Cui, C., Li, Y., Geng, D., Zhang, H., & Jin, C. (2018). The effectiveness of evidence-based nursing on development of nursing students' critical thinking: A meta-analysis. *Nurse Education Today, 65*, 46–53. doi:https://doi.org/10.1016/j.nedt.2018.02.036

Culyer, L. M., Jatulis, L. L., Cannistraci, P., & Brownell, C. A. (2018). Evidenced-based teaching strategies that facilitate transfer of knowledge between theory and practice: What are nursing faculty using? *Teaching & Learning in Nursing, 13*(3), 174–179. doi:10.1016/j.teln.2018.03.003

Dwyer, P. A., & Revell, S. M. H. (2015). Preparing students for the emotional challenges of nursing: An integrative review. *Journal of Nursing Education, 54*(1), 7–12+sup. doi:10.3928/01484834-20141224-06

Emerson, R. J., & Records, K. (2008). Today's challenge, tomorrow's excellence: The practice of evidence-based education. *Journal of Nursing Education, 47*(8), 359–370. Retrieved from http://search.proquest.com/docview/203964999?accountid=100

Frenn, M., & Dreifuerst, K. (2018). Summary of research using the NLN Core Competencies as a framework. In J. A. Halstead (Ed.), *Nurse educator competencies: Creating an evidence based practice for nurse educators* (2nd ed.). Alphen aan den Rijn, Netherlands: Wolters Kluwer.

Frenn, M., & Dreifuerst, K. T. (2019). Summary of research using the NLN Core Competencies as a framework. In J. A. Halstead (Ed.), *NLN core competencies for nurse educators: A decade of influence* (2nd ed.). Philadelphia, PA: Wolters Kluwer.

Garner, S. L., Killingsworth, E., Bradshaw, M., Raj, L., Johnson, S. R., Abijah, S. P., . . . Victor, S. (2018). The impact of simulation education on self-efficacy towards teaching for nurse educators. *International Nursing Review, 65*(4), 586–595. doi:10.1111/inr.12455

Gresley, R. S. (2009). Building a science of nursing education. In C.M. Schultz (Ed.). *Building a science of nursing education: Foundation for evidence-based teaching-learning* (pp.1–13). New York: National League for Nursing.

Halstead, J. (2007). *Nurse educator competencies: Creating an evidence-based practice for nurse educators*. New York, NY: National League for Nursing.

Halstead, J. A. (2019). *NLN core competencies for nurse educators: A decade of influence*. Philadelphia, PA: Wolters Kluwer.

Health Evidence. (2013). Quality assessment tool—Review articles. Retrieved from https://www.healthevidence.org/documents/our-appraisal-tools/QA_tool&dictionary_18.Mar.2013.pdf

Hutchings, P., Huber, M. T., & Ciccone, A. (2011). *The scholarship of teaching and learning reconsidered: Institutional integration and impact*. San Francisco, CA: Jossey-Bass.

Im, E.-O., & Chang, S. J. (2012). A systematic integrated literature review of systematic integrated literature reviews in nursing. *Journal of Nursing Education, 51*, 632–645.

Institute of Medicine. (2010). *The future of nursing: Leading change, advancing health*. Washington, DC: National Academies Press.

Interprofessional Education Collaborative. (2016). Core Competencies for Interprofessional Collaborative Practice: 2016 Update. Retrieved from https://hsc.unm.edu/ipe/resources/ipec-2016-core-competencies.pdf

Kalb, K. A., O'Conner-Von, S. K., Brockway, C., Rierson, C. L., & Sendelbach, S. (2015). Evidence-based teaching practice in nursing education: Faculty perspectives and practices. *Nursing Education Perspectives, 36*(4), 212–219. doi:10.5480/14-1472

Kragelund, L. (2013). The obser-view: A method of generating data and learning. *Nurse Researcher, 20*(5), 6–10.

Landeen, J., Carr, D., Culver, K., Martin, L., Matthew-Maich, N., Noesgaard, C., & Beney-Gadsby, L. (2016). The impact of curricular changes on BSCN students' clinical learning outcomes. *Nurse Education in Practice, 21*, 51–58. doi:10.1016/j.nepr.2016.09.010

Levey, J. A. (2018). Universal Design for Instruction in nursing education: An integrative review. *Nursing Education Perspectives, 39*(3), 156–161. doi:10.1097/01. NEP.0000000000000249

Limoges, J., & Acorn, S. (2016). Transforming practice into clinical scholarship. *Journal of Advanced Nursing, 72*(4), 747–753. doi:10.1111/jan.12881

Melnyk, B. M., Fineout-Overholt, E., Gallagher-Ford, L., & Kaplan, L. (2012). The state of evidence-based practice in US nurses: Critical implications for nurse leaders and education. *Journal of Nursing Administration, 42*, 410–417.

Miller, J. J., Grise-Owens, E., Drury, W., & Rickman, C. (2018). Teaching note—Developing a professional writing course using a holistic view of competence. *Journal of Social Work Education, 54*(4), 709–714. doi:10.1080/10437797.2018.1474152

Morin, K. (2012). Fostering rigorous critique of the evidence. *Journal of Nursing Education, 51*, 663–664. doi: 10.3928/01484834-20121119-01

National League for Nursing. (2016). NLN research priorities in nursing education 2016–2019. Retrieved from http://www.nln.org/docs/default-source/professional-development-programs/nln-research-priorities-in-nursing-education-single-pages.pdf?sfvrsn=2

National League for Nursing. (2019a). Core values. Retrieved from http://www.nln.org/about/core-values

National League for Nursing. (2019b). NLN Chamberlain University College of Nursing Center for the Advancement of the Science of Nursing Education. Retrieved from http://www.nln.org/centers-for-nursing-education/nln-chamberlain-university-college-of-nursing-center-for-the-advancement-of-the-science-of-nursing-education2

Njie-Carr, V. P. S., Ludeman, E., Mei Ching, L. E. E., Dordunoo, D., Trocky, N. M., & Jenkins, L. S. (2017). An integrative review of flipped classroom teaching models in nursing education. *Journal of Professional Nursing, 33*(2), 133–144. doi:10.1016/j.profnurs.2016.07.001

Nosek, C. M., Scheckel, M. M., Waterbury, T., Macdonald, A. N. N., & Wozney, N. (2017). The Collaborative Improvement Model: An interpretive study of revising a curriculum. *Journal of Professional Nursing, 33*(1), 38–50. doi:10.1016/j.profnurs.2016.05.006

Oermann, M. H. (2009). Evidence-based programs and teaching/evaluation methods: Needed to achieve excellence in nursing education. In M. H. Adams, & T. M. Valiga (Eds.), *Achieving excellence in nursing education* (pp. 63–76). New York, NY: National League for Nursing.

Oermann, M. H. (2017). From the editor. Building your scholarship from your teaching: Plan now. *Nurse Educator, 42*(5), 217. doi:10.1097/NNE.0000000000000417

Oermann, M. H. (2018). Wanted: Evidence to guide clinical teaching. *Nurse Educator, 43*(5), 223. doi:10.1097/NNE.0000000000000594

Patterson, B., Billings, D. M., Halstead, J. A., Yoder-Wise, P. S., Fitzpatrick, J., Morin, K. H., & Oermann, M. H. (2018). Letter to the editor.... Morton, P. Nursing education research: An editor's view. *Journal of Professional Nursing, 2017;33*:311–312. *Journal of Professional Nursing, 34*(3), 157–158. doi:10.1016/j.profnurs.2018.01.003

Patterson, B. J., & McLaughlin, K. (2019). Competency VII: Engage in scholarship. In J. A. Halstead (Ed.), *NLN core competencies for nurse educators: A decade of influence.* Philadelphia, PA: Wolters Kluwer.

Polit, D. F., & Beck, C. T. (2017). *Nursing research: Generating and assessing evidence for nursing practice* (10th ed.). Philadelphia: Wolters Kluwer.

Raymond, C., Profetto-McGrath, J., Myrick, F., & Strean, W. B. (2018). Process matters: Successes and challenges of recruiting and retaining participants for nursing education research. *Nurse Educator, 43*(2), 92–96. doi:10.1097/NNE.0000000000000423

Rozelle, C. (2018). Exposing students to diverse health care teams. *ABNF Journal, 29*(1), 5–7.

Shulman, L. S. (2008). Foreword. In G. E. Walker, C. M. Golde, L. Jones, A. Conkline Bueschel, & P. Hutchings. *The formation of scholars: Rethinking doctoral education for the twenty-first century.* San Francisco, CA: Jossey Bass.

Simons, T. L. (1999). Behavioral integrity as a critical ingredient for transformational leadership. *Journal of Organizational Change Management, 12*(2), 89–104.

Smith, M. H. (2012). *The legal, professional, and ethical dimensions of education in nursing.* New York, NY: Springer.

Speakman, E. (2016). *Interprofessional education and collaborative practice: Creating a blueprint for nurse educators.* Washington, D.C.: The National League for Nursing.

Spurlock, D. R. (2017). Measurement matters: Improving measurement practices in nursing education research. *Journal of Nursing Education, 56*(5), 257–259. doi:10.3928/01484834-20170424-01

Spurlock, D. R. (2018a). The single-group, pre- and posttest design in nursing education research: It's time to move on. *Journal of Nursing Education, 57*(2), 69–71. doi:10.3928/01484834-20180123-02

Spurlock, D. R. (2018b). What's in a name? Revisiting pilot studies in nursing education research. *Journal of Nursing Education, 57*(8), 457–459. doi:10.3928/01484834-20180720-02

Spurlock Jr., D. (2017). Beyond p < .05: Toward a Nightingalean perspective on statistical significance for nursing education researchers. *Journal of Nursing Education, 56*(8), 453–455. doi:10.3928/01484834-20170712-02

Stephens, T. M., & Gunther, M. E. (2016). Twitter, millennials, and nursing education research. *Nursing Education Perspectives, 37*(1), 23–27. doi:10.5480/14-1462

Taylor, J., & Spurlock, D. (2018). Statistical power in nursing education research. *Journal of Nursing Education, 57*(5), 262–264. doi:10.3928/01484834-20180420-02

Van Der Like, J. J., Fox, H., Blackburn, A., & Chisholm, J. (2019). Advocating for mental health nursing care education using a flipped classroom. *Creative Nursing*, 25(1), 32–37. doi:10.1891/1078-4535.25.1.32

VanGraafeiland, B., Sloand, E., Silbert-Flagg, J., Gleason, K., & Dennison Himmelfarb, C. (2019). Academic-clinical service partnerships are innovative strategies to advance patient safety competence and leadership in prelicensure nursing students. *Nursing Outlook*, 67(1), 49–53. doi:10.1016/j.outlook.2018.08.003

Weaver, A. J., Haak, N. J., Molt, L., & Cannon, A. R. (2018). Let's do the twist: Pairing interdisciplinary collaborative teaching, and hands-on and service learning opportunities, to spread awareness of communication sciences and disorders. *Perspectives of the ASHA Special Interest Groups*, 3(10), 27–44. doi:10.1044/persp3.SIG10.27

Wesp, L. M., Scheer, V., Ruiz, A., Walker, K., Weitzel, J., Shaw, L., … Mkandawire-Valhmu, L. (2018). An emancipatory approach to cultural competency: The application of critical race, postcolonial, and intersectionality theories. *Advances in Nursing Science*, 41(4), 316–326. doi:10.1097/ANS.0000000000000230

Whittemore, R. & Knafl, K. (2005). The integrative review: Updated methodology. *Journal of Advanced Nursing*, 52(5), 546–553. doi: 10.1111/j.1365-2648.2005.03621.x

World Health Organization. (2016). *Nurse educator core competencies*. Retrieved from https://www.who.int/hrh/nursing_midwifery/nurse_educator050416.pdf

Yue, M., Zhang, M., Zhang, C., & Jin, C. (2017). The effectiveness of concept mapping on development of critical thinking in nursing education: A systematic review and meta-analysis. *Nurse Education Today*, 52, 87–94. doi:https://doi.org/10.1016/j.nedt.2017.02.018

Function Effectively within the Organizational Environment and the Academic Community

Nancy C. Sharts-Hopko, PhD, RN, CNE, ANEF, FAAN

The CNE Test Plan lists the following for the area of Function Effectively within the Organizational Environment and the Academic Community:

C. Function Effectively within the Organizational Environment and the Academic Community

1. Identify how social, economic, political, and institutional forces influence nursing and higher education.
2. Make decisions based on knowledge of historical and current trends and issues in higher education.
3. Integrate the values of respect, collegiality, professionalism, and caring to build an organizational climate that fosters the development of learners and colleagues.
4. Consider the goals of the nursing program and the mission of the parent institution when proposing change or managing issues.
5. Participate on institutional and departmental committees.

These activities are noted in the detailed CNE® test blueprint for Category 6C (National League for Nursing [NLN], 2018). They reflect the role of the nurse educator within the academic organization and community. The five major areas identified in the blueprint are critical to nurse educators' successful navigation of the work organization, and each will be addressed in this chapter.

OVERVIEW

Nurses who assume academic positions typically observe striking differences between the culture of higher education and the culture of health care delivery. Successful nurse educators are attuned not only to effective design and implementation of programs that promote students' mastery of professional competencies but also to the environment of their academic institution as well as the sociopolitical and economic context of higher education in which it operates. While both types of organizations respond to accreditation standards reflecting current professional evidence-based consensus on quality, differences are marked, as presented in Table 8.1 (Zemsky, 2013).

Table 8.1

Cultural Differences Between Health Care and Higher Education Organizations

Health Care Organizations	Higher Education Organizations
• Bottom-line focus on metrics-driven policies, practices • Focus on patient/population outcomes • Change is rapid, reflecting cash flow, patient outcomes • Employees' continuation is performance based and related to changing organizational needs	• Focus on organizational outcomes just beginning to permeate academic units in higher education • Focus on student growth • Change can be slow, related to faculty autonomy and governance • Employees may be permanently contracted (tenured)

Effective functioning in an academic environment requires nurse educators to be conversant with historical and current trends in higher education and nursing education, to develop effective vertical and horizontal collaborations throughout the educational institution, to balance professional and institutional expectations individually and in terms of the nursing unit, and to engage in institutional leadership as well as advocacy for the unique characteristics of the discipline of nursing (NLN, 2012).

A universal challenge for nursing faculty is their ability to balance maintenance of clinical expertise with typical academic expectations regarding teaching, scholarship, and institutional and professional service. In addition, the nature of clinical instruction is that it is labor intensive, therefore expensive, requiring faculty to be absent from the academic institution for significant periods of time. These factors require constant interpretation of the nurse faculty role to other colleagues and administrators.

IDENTIFY HOW SOCIAL, ECONOMIC, POLITICAL, AND INSTITUTIONAL FORCES INFLUENCE NURSING AND HIGHER EDUCATION

Table 8.2 identifies some key milestones in the evolution of nursing education in the United States (Keeling, 2017; Meleis, 2018). This very brief rendition of our history illustrates a progression from establishment of the structure for nursing education to focus on educational quality and patient-care outcomes.

Nurse educators need to be aware of the organizational context in which they teach. Schools of nursing may be freestanding or in health professions educational institutions in association with health care systems. As such, they may offer a diploma as well as associate, bachelor, master's, Doctor of Nursing Practice, or PhD degrees. Alternatively, they may be located in traditional colleges or universities that are broadly classified as associate, bachelor, master's, doctoral, or research-intensive institutions (Carnegie Classification of Institutions of Higher Education, 2019). In addition, institutions may be identified as public, private secular, or private religious; not for profit or proprietary; and virtual (online) or campus-based.

It is critical that nurses understand the types of faculty appointments represented in their organization. Major types of faculty appointments are depicted in Table 8.3 (American Association of University Professors, 2014).

Table 8.2

Key Milestones in the Evolution of Nursing Education in the United States

Date	Milestone(s)
1860	Florence Nightingale launched the Nightingale Training School at St. Thomas's Hospital, London.
Late 19th to early 20th century	Nightingale schools proliferated in the United States.
1900	Adelaide Nutting and Isobel Hampton Robb introduced a program for nursing teachers at Teachers College of Columbia University in New York City.
1923	The Goldmark Report recommended standards for nursing education; the Rockefeller Foundation established the first autonomous academic nursing unit at Yale University.
1934	New York University offered the first doctoral degree in nursing.
World War II	70,000 nurse veterans become eligible for the GI Bill and entered universities.
1948	The Brown Report urged the movement of nursing education into colleges/universities.
1952	The National League for Nursing began to accredit schools of nursing.
1965	The American Nurses Association endorsed BSN entry into professional nursing. The first program to train nurse practitioners begins at the University of Colorado.
1970	The National Commission on Nursing and Nursing Education (Lysaught Report) endorsed BSN entry into nursing and graduate preparation of faculty.
1986	The National Center for Nursing Research (later, the National Institute for Nursing Research) is established at the National Institutes of Health.
1999	University of Tennessee Health Science Center launched the first DNP program.
2010	The Institute of Medicine report on the Future of Nursing recommended nurses practice at the highest level of preparation, and recommended more nurses prepared for doctorates to address the nation's health needs

Table 8.3

Major Types of Faculty Appointments

Type of Faculty Appointment	Description
Adjunct	Part-time status on a per-course basis (clinical or classroom based); includes clinical instructors.
Contingent or nontenure track	Full-time status for teaching or service but typically not scholarship. Contracts are 1 year in duration and over time may extend to renewable periods of 3, 5, or more years.
Tenure track	A probationary period during which the faculty member demonstrates progress in accordance with institutional standards in teaching, scholarship, and institutional/professional service.
Tenure	A permanent appointment until retirement.

Full-time faculty may be ranked, commonly as instructor, assistant professor, associate professor, or professor. The rank of emeritus is bestowed on retired faculty who have served with distinction. Additionally, nurse educators can encounter a wide range of academic expectations about how many months an annual contract covers, how many teaching credits they are required to assume in a year, and much time they are required to spend at the institution, even within an individual school. It is important to ask specifically about the requirements of one's own academic appointment.

Scenario 8.1

Four new faculty members were recently hired in the Department of Nursing in a private university that does not have a collective bargaining unit. Two of the four have complained to their department chairperson that they seem to carry far greater teaching loads than the other two. The practice in this institution is to treat contracts as private information, individually negotiated with the department chairperson.

The department chairperson has pointed out they are contingent, or nontenure-track, faculty. The other two people whose workloads they are comparing to their own are tenure-track faculty.

Consider:
1. Based on the information that is provided, do the two complainants actually know what their colleagues' workloads are?
2. What change in institutional practice could alleviate such perceptions and complaints?
3. What usual expectations of the tenure-track faculty could account for differences in teaching and service assignments?
4. What do you know from the information that is provided about practice requirements for this group of faculty?
5. What would you recommend the chairperson do to address this discord in the department?

In the United States, accrediting bodies generally require that educators of registered nurses hold a graduate degree in nursing (Accreditation Commission for Nursing Education [ACEN], 2019; Commission on Collegiate Nursing Education [CCNE], 2018; Commission for Nursing Education Accreditation [CNEA], 2019). Many institutions require that faculty hold a terminal degree, typically a doctorate, for appointment to the tenure track. Within the past decade, nurses graduating with the Doctor of Nursing Practice (DNP) credential have far outnumbered nurses graduating with a research doctorate (typically a PhD). While the DNP was created to prepare leaders for transformation in health care delivery (American Association of Colleges of Nursing [AACN], 2006), a significant portion of DNP graduates enter academia (Fang & Bednash, 2017). This has led to concerns related to DNP graduates' ability to satisfy requirements for tenure, particularly in the area of scholarship, in academic institutions where tenure decisions rest with committees comprising mostly nonnursing faculty. This debate is occurring against a backdrop of a severe and worsening shortage of nursing faculty in the United States and elsewhere (AACN, 2017).

Nurse educators will be well served to understand institutions' mission and heritage as they consider where to teach and then how to thrive in their institution after joining the faculty. Box 8.1 depicts important mission-related differences among institutions that shape expectations for faculty.

BOX 8.1 Mission-Related Differences Among Institutions of Higher Learning
• Publicly versus privately funded institution
• Population primarily served (e.g., undergraduate vs. graduate; demographic make-up of student population)
• Philosophical/religious orientation
• Primary education focus (e.g., science, technology, engineering, and mathematics [STEM] versus liberal arts)
• How scholarly productivity is defined (e.g., priority on federally funded research)
• Key external partnerships and stakeholders

MAKE DECISIONS BASED ON KNOWLEDGE OF HISTORICAL AND CURRENT TRENDS AND ISSUES IN HIGHER EDUCATION

Since the early 20th century, nursing organizations have generated standards for ensuring quality in nursing education (National League of Nursing Education, 1937). Today, three organizations are authorized by the United States Department of Education to accredit nursing programs in general. In addition, an American Association of Nurse Anesthetists subsidiary accredits nurse anesthesia programs, while the American Nurses Association entity, the American Nurses Credentialing Center, accredits programs of continuing education. These accrediting bodies are described in Table 8.4.

Each accrediting body issues curricular requirements and standards for the overall organization of the academic unit, sufficiency of resources, qualifications of faculty, and monitoring of program outcomes. An academic unit will likely maintain general academic program accreditation, though it is voluntary. Some programs opt out of accreditation; however, this restricts financial aid opportunities for their students and some career paths for graduates. In addition to general program accreditation, a school may also pursue accreditation of a nurse anesthesia program and a continuing education program. Each accreditation requires periodic self-study, peer visitation, and review on a regular basis.

Table 8.4

Accrediting Bodies in Nursing Education

Accrediting Body	Description
Accreditation Commission for Nursing Education	Accredits LPN through DNP and certificate programs.
Collegiate Commission on Nursing Education	Subsidiary of the American Association of Colleges of Nursing; accredits baccalaureate and higher-degree as well as post-MSN APRN programs
Commission for Nursing Education Accreditation	Subsidiary of the National League for Nursing; accredits LPN through DNP programs.
Commission on Accreditation of Nurse Anesthesia Educational Programs	Subsidiary of the American Association of Nurse Anesthetists; accredits nurse anesthetists.
American Nurses Credentialing Center	Subsidiary of the American Nurses Association; accredits providers of continuing education.

BOX 8.2 Key Current Issues Influencing Nursing Education
• Growing demand for nurses/health care services as baby boomers age and more people access services • Crisis of student debt • Financial strain on colleges and universities • Urgency of improving safety/quality in health care • Growing integration of technology in health care • Increased recognition of unique needs of vulnerable populations • Globalization

In addition to accreditation of the nursing unit, it is the responsibility of nurse educators to participate in the process of obtaining and maintaining other accreditations sought by their employing organization. This may include whole-institution accreditation from one of the seven regional accrediting commissions within the Council of Regional Accrediting Commissions (C-RAC) (C-RAC, 2019). These organizations are authorized by the U.S. Department of Education to accredit schools. Accreditation is important for federal benefits, including students' access to federally guaranteed loans. Nurse educators may also participate in accreditation for specialized nonacademic units of their institution, including, for example, the National Collegiate Athletic Association (NCAA).

Box 8.2 identities key current issues that bear on nursing education. Collectively, these issues impact both what we teach and how we teach. After publication of the 2010 Institute of Medicine (IOM) report, *The Future of Nursing: Leading Change, Advancing Health,* nurse educators have worked to implement two specific recommendations about the education of nurses in response to the national capacity to ensure care for the public:

1. that the percentage of bachelor's degree prepared nurses reaches 80 percent by 2020, and
2. that the number of nurses prepared for doctorates doubles by that year.

Interim reporting in 2018 (Lippincott Solutions, 2018) indicated that the proportion of registered nurses with a BSN had increased from 49 percent in 2010 to 54 percent by 2016; thus, efforts must continue to bring the nursing labor force to the 80 percent BSN-prepared goal. Meanwhile, the number of nurses prepared for doctorates had more than doubled, to 22,454, though the marked tilt toward DNP preparation was an unexpected outcome whose effects are unknown.

The high cost of higher education is generating tremendous upheaval institutionally and among policy makers. Over the past 30 years, the cost of a college education has increased at a rate far steeper than the Consumer Price Index (College Board, 2019). Public institutions have experienced reduced support from their states, and students across all types of institutions have borrowed heavily to finance their education. College graduates' burden of debt is a major concern for the U.S. Department of Education and elected representatives. Academic institutions are increasingly being held accountable to ensure that students can complete programs and become employed so that they are better off, rather than worse off, for having attended college.

Despite academic institutions intensifying attention on operating as cost-effectively as possible, the rate of schools closing has increased markedly in recent years. Several studies have predicted an acceleration in the rate at which American colleges and universities close due to financial stress (Lindsay, 2015). Some faculty in public institutions have been required to take furloughs, increase their teaching loads, or accept reductions in salary (Filby, 2019). According to Lindsay, private institutions are particularly vulnerable to closure.

Among the various academic units in higher education, nursing education is fortunate that the prospects for the employability of graduates is strong as Baby Boomer era nurses retire, as more previously uninsured people are enabled to access health care, and as a growing cadre of older adults require health services. The Bureau of Labor Statistics (2018) predicts a 15 percent growth in registered nurse jobs by 2026. Because nursing is an attractive major with good career prospects, some educational institutions seek to shore up revenue by aggressively expanding nursing programs, which can strain the nursing unit's human and physical resources.

At this writing, medical error has become the third leading cause of death in the United States (Makary & Daniel, 2016). The IOM has sounded the alert about patient safety since publication of its 1999 report, *To Err is Human*. From this awareness, nurse educators responded with the development of the Quality and Safety Education for Nurses (QSEN) project (QSEN Institute, 2019), which offers training to promote educational standards related to patient safety, threading quality throughout curricula to nurse educators, and relevant teaching strategies.

Concern with patient safety has also fueled myriad educational innovations to promote better interprofessional communication. Interprofessional education is intended to promote effective functioning of health care teams by leveling intrateam hierarchies, enhancing communication, and promoting the norm that any team member can identify a potential error before it occurs (Brook et al., 2013). Not all schools of nursing have the opportunity to collaborate with students majoring in other health professions. This trend has forced programs to consider potential educational partnerships with faculty in schools of law, business, and engineering, or programs in ethics to develop learning or service opportunities that are potentially enriching and meaningful for all student participants. Collaboratives across institutions also have emerged.

Scenario 8.2

The university has a learning outcome that all baccalaureate graduates will demonstrate proficiency in the use of technology to access and evaluate information and manage data. For nearly a decade, the Department of Nursing has implemented a policy that discouraged student use of social media and apps of any kind. Meanwhile, other health professions, computing, and engineering departments within the university are promoting the integration of technology into students' clinical experiences, including the development of social media strategies and apps to promote patients' health in clinical practice. The nursing faculty are divided over the appropriateness of the use of technology in clinical settings.

Consider:
1. What information will be useful for the nursing faculty to consider as they determine how to strengthen their program in relation to this university learning outcome?
2. What partnerships within the university would be useful for the nursing faculty to develop as they begin to move in this area?
3. What community and university resources are available to them as they think about their policies?
4. What are the most important principles to address in regard to responsible use of technology in patient care settings?
5. What strategies can be devised to ensure that faculty have the facility with technology that they need?

Technological innovations—for example, high-fidelity simulators and response clickers or smartphone applications—have permeated clinical laboratories and classrooms. It is now widely recognized that the growing domains of robotics technology and social media have much to offer in educating nursing students as well as patients and fostering patients' independence. Nurse educators are challenged not only to develop technological proficiency comparable to their Millennial students but also to develop the expertise and insight to offer guidance about critical assessment of these ever-emerging tools. Additionally, electronic health records (EHRs) are still in their infancy; we can envision a future in which user-friendly, seamless EHRs truly support quality in health care as well as real-time, evidence-based decision-making.

In addition to greater inclusion of previously uninsured populations and a shift in the locus of care, new recognition of populations with particular issues—such as veterans returning from the Iraq and Afghan wars—represents a challenge to nurse educators as they prepare students to interact with patients holistically and recognize their unique needs (Marion et al., 2016). Additional examples of historical events that provoked nurse educators to reevaluate how curricula addressed specific population needs include Hurricane Katrina in 2005 and current international concerns about how the effects of global warming on the environment may affect population health. Yet another example of increasing recognition of an area of diversity that requires particular attention in the delivery of health care and in higher education is the range of gender identity that students as well as patients express. Schools are increasingly aware of needs for accommodations, such as gender-neutral restrooms, consideration in housing assignments, athletic team eligibility, and eligibility to attend single-sex colleges (Gardner, 2015).

Scenario 8.3

A small public university is located in a rural, socially conservative part of its state. The Department of Nursing embraces all relevant professional standards. At the same time, the local practice settings, both public and private, maintain traditional policies. A nursing student who is currently in clinical rotations has revealed to the academic adviser that she is transgender and will begin publicly presenting as male. The adviser consults with the department chair because the adviser is concerned that the student may be exposed to incivility within the department and that this may be an issue with the clinical partners.

Consider:
1. What information should the department chair obtain as the chair begins to think about this student's rights?
2. Who are the stakeholders in this situation?
3. What rights of this student, other students, and patients bear on this situation?
4. What conversation should happen between the adviser, department chair, and student?
5. What resources might be useful for the student, faculty, and administration within the institution and the community?
6. By what criteria should the student be evaluated?
7. How might the department chair approach clinical partners regarding students representing diverse populations in general and this student in particular?

One additional trend that bears discussion is the increasing recognition by nurse educators that students must be prepared to consider health globally even if they practice in a geographically circumscribed area. Throughout their careers, students will encounter patients and colleagues from around the world, and they will look beyond national borders for solutions to our most intractable health care problems. Many schools of nursing now offer some students international immersion experiences. In addition to gaining appreciation for the interplay among culture, geography, and health, an additional learning outcome is the ability to compare differing health care delivery systems. In a time of growing concern about climate change, air travel is associated with significant emissions (International Civil Aviation Organization, 2019). Nurse educators are challenged to determine the most efficient and cost-effective, as well as environmentally neutral, way to ensure that all students can develop competence in the area of culture and global health (Spector, 2016).

INTEGRATE THE VALUES OF RESPECT, COLLEGIALITY, PROFESSIONALISM, AND CARING TO BUILD AN ORGANIZATIONAL CLIMATE THAT FOSTERS THE DEVELOPMENT OF LEARNERS AND COLLEAGUES

Academic institutions are hierarchical entities with traditions and norms that date back to their medieval origins. Incivility in academic environments has emerged as a concern that threatens the quality of students' educational experience. Incivility, lateral violence, and bullying behavior occur within and across all levels of people in academic institutions: administrators, faculty, staff, and students (Perry & Blincoe, 2015). Both lateral violence and faculty bullying of students are topics that have received considerable attention in the nursing education literature (Milesky, Baptiste, Foronda, Dupler, & Belcher, 2015). Box 8.3 identifies characteristics that place universities at risk for incivility (Hollis, 2015).

Incivility matters because it is costly in terms of lost productivity and diminished teaching effectiveness, diminished retention of student and faculty talent, legal risk, and the psychological toll on observers as well as victims (Lester, 2013). In contrast, an organizational culture of appreciation is associated with increased productivity and satisfaction, creativity and innovation, and positive socialization of students and junior faculty. The tone must be set at the top of the organization.

At times, a commitment to academic freedom has been used to cloak incivility. In general, academic freedom refers to faculty members' expertise in regard to their content and self-determination regarding methods by which they teach; their freedom to determine their topic and methods of research in their discipline; and their right to control curricula in their discipline, admission standards for students, and standards for the evaluation of peers for employment, tenure, and

---

BOX 8.3 Organizational Factors that Increase the Risk of Fostering Incivility in Academic Institutions

- Strict hierarchy of ranks
- Organizational change
- Management lacking authority
- Poorly organized work
- Workloads that are individually negotiated
- Role conflict
- Conflicting goals
- High job insecurity
- Subjective performance measures
- Competitive, individualistic nature of faculty work
- Shrinking resources

promotion. The American Association of University Professors (AAUP) is explicitly clear that academic freedom is not an endorsement of hate speech or uncivil behavior (Reichman, 2017).

An institutional commitment to recruitment of students and employees for diversity and inclusion aims to ensure that students are well prepared to prosper in a pluralistic society. Building on the civil rights and women's movements of the 1970s on racial and ethnic inclusion and parity for women, efforts are now expanding in higher education to consider the vantage point of persons representing many types of otherness, including persons with disabilities, first-generation college attendees, veterans, nonbinary gender identities, country of origin, and immigrant status. For example, holistic admission practices for students are linked to the institutional mission and values, placing priority on diversity. Qualitative data are considered while reducing reliance on standardized examination scores. Specifically, all people who meet eligibility requirements are deemed admissible rather than simply admitting the desired number starting with the top scorer and moving down a numerically ordered list (AACN, 2019).

Students and junior faculty representing diverse or educationally underserved populations may have little familiarity with educational norms in colleges and universities. They require institutional resources to ensure that they are able to capitalize on their potential to succeed. These may include formal and informal peer mentoring, tutoring, advising, coaching, and other forms of social as well as academic support (Gregory & Chapman, 2012).

CONSIDER THE GOALS OF THE NURSING PROGRAM AND THE MISSION OF THE PARENT INSTITUTION WHEN PROPOSING CHANGE OR MANAGING ISSUES

Academic programs need to further the overall mission of the institution in which they reside. In colleges and universities, the academic nursing unit is likely to function with a higher degree of multidisciplinary collaboration than in a freestanding nursing or health professions educational institution. This requires understanding of how the nursing unit in the institution articulates with other parts of the organization as well as external entities. Box 8.4 depicts relevant considerations related to organizational structure and lines of authority for nurse educators.

Undergraduate nursing programs in particular may be expected to incorporate a core common to all undergraduate students that aligns with the overall mission, heritage, and values of the institution. For example, a religiously affiliated college may have an unusually significant requirement in religious studies, philosophy, and ethics. All students in the institution, no matter their major, may be required to participate in an international immersion experience. There may be

---

BOX 8.4 Internal and External Authority Over Nursing Unit Function

- What is the chain of authority from the head of the nursing unit to the president of the institution?
- To whom does the president report?
- What are the areas of the institution headed by vice presidents, and how does the nursing unit relate to them?
- How and by whom is the institutional budget approved?
- What external entities exercise direct control over the institution, for example, government structures, shareholders, or religious organizations?

a service-learning requirement in addition to the nursing practica. Students may be required to fulfill requirements in writing, numeracy, cultural diversity, civics, fine arts, foreign languages, or even swimming. Faculty in baccalaureate as well as graduate programs in more research-intensive environments may be urged to increase the opportunity for individual student research. It becomes a challenge for nurse educators to design academic programs that respond sufficiently to both institutional mission-driven as well as professional requirements. To keep the nursing program within a reasonable total of credits, faculty will find themselves debating how to exchange old curriculum content for new additions. Nurse educators may be assisted in their work by the opportunity to participate in faculty development workshops that foster their appreciation of values that are central to their institution.

In terms of managing groups of faculty, nursing academic administrators are mindful of the expectations of an individual institution as they assign teaching and advise faculty members about time management in relation to the expectations of their appointments. In a teaching-focused institution, there is a fairly high degree of consistency in how faculty members perceive their roles and how teaching assignments are distributed. Faculty may have time dedicated to their own clinical practice, some faculty may have their teaching loads reduced for administrative responsibilities, and faculty members will support their own academic unit as well as the larger institution through committee work. But in general, faculty members in these organizations understand that they are all there to implement the curriculum.

As institutions become more heavily focused on graduate education, and particularly on research, the expectations become more diverse. Graduate faculty may have teaching assignments that include less direct clinical supervision or classroom instruction and more individual mentoring of students. Individual mentoring may not appear on teaching schedules, and their loads may appear to be much lighter than those of the undergraduate faculty. Faculty with research expectations may have substantial teaching load reductions at times, for instance, prior to tenure; this can seem unfair to nontenure track faculty or to older tenured faculty who did not have such an advantage when they were new faculty. Faculty with funding for research may be able to buy out most of their teaching time, but they will face expectations to mentor students or junior faculty in research and to produce and publish results within a specified time frame that may also include writing the next grants to continue their work. Transparency about who is doing what and the expectations that all faculty face, along with open dialogue for meeting the academic unit's goals, can go a long way toward ameliorating perceptions of unfairness (Flaherty, 2019).

Academic administrators are increasingly focused on the generation of funds to support students financially, to support the costs of their more traditional programs, and to fund the expensive technology that is increasingly required to ensure students' competence, such as simulation labs. Fundraising may come from submission of grants for program development, facilities, or equipment; research grants that pay overhead to the school; solicitation of donations from alumni and philanthropists interested in nursing; and the development of profit-bearing academic and nonacademic programs (Council for the Advancement and Support of Education, 2019).

One challenge for nursing faculty that was alluded to previously is that clinical practice may or may not be regarded by the institution as a component of the faculty role. In some institutions, nurse faculty practice is regarded as competitive with full-time employment by the institution, and they may need to apply for special permission to engage in it, though some nursing education administrators have been successful in negotiating recognition for faculty practice. This can be a particularly challenging dilemma for faculty members whose certifications require a significant amount of clinical practice and who are employed to teach in a track that requires them to maintain certification (AAUP, 2006). In some institutions, faculty members who teach in advanced practice programs are ineligible for the tenure track because of their substantial practice requirements.

Institutions of higher education often have an interest in the development of the student as a whole person. Faculty members may be called on to interact with students in capacities beyond formal teaching and advising, and they may find it enlightening as well as rewarding to interact with students outside of the nursing major. Opportunities may involve such activities as co-curricular learning interactions, participation in volunteer service, or faculty sponsorship of a student organization or activity. Students gain from the opportunity to relate to faculty outside their formal roles, and these can be ways to encourage students in all disciplines to consider careers in higher education.

PARTICIPATE ON INSTITUTIONAL AND DEPARTMENTAL COMMITTEES

Nurse educators are well served to know how the nursing unit fits into the overall organizational chart of the institution as well as who are the top-level administrators and members of the board of trustees (see Box 8.4). It is strategic to know some of the important accomplishments in various academic and nonacademic units, as faculty members represent their institutions as a whole in the local community and through their professional activities and will be asked about these matters.

It is important to take advantage of opportunities to interact with institutional leaders and colleagues at all levels across the institution for several reasons. Research indicates that women faculty members, the majority of nurse educators, tend to give less time and attention to business-related social interactions to the detriment of their advancement in the college or university (*Chronicle of Higher Education*, 2018). It can be extremely important when a faculty member seeks tenure or promotion to be known by deans, tenure committee members, and administrators who will be making the decision on their behalf. Moreover, when a nursing faculty member is engaged in a matter that relates to, or requires assistance from, others in the system—for example, seeking to change the way a nonnursing course in the nursing curriculum is being taught—it is invaluable to have relationships with people prior to seeking their help. Interactions with academic colleagues throughout the institution may lead to ideas for interprofessional courses, service-learning activities, or research projects. Moreover, it is extremely enlightening to learn about the organization through the eyes of people outside of one's own discipline. For some institutional activities, attendance is mandatory and, by all means, faculty members must be attentive to those expectations. Even if they are not required to attend, however, it is wise to participate.

As mentioned earlier, faculty at some institutions are members of organized labor units and engage in collective bargaining related to the terms of their contracts. Faculty members who are at a unionized institution need to understand what it means to join the union or not join, as well as the issues under discussion and the political costs and benefits of being actively engaged in advocacy related to their contracts at various stages of their careers. Specifically, it may be unwise for a tenure-track faculty member to run for office in the collective bargaining unit. After tenure, however, a faculty member can offer the perspective of time in the institution with little risk.

Most higher education institutions have a structure for faculty governance, such as a faculty senate, and a way for faculty members to be represented on major committees of the institution. These can include, for example, the committee for tenure and promotion, committees related to salary and benefits, search committees for administrative positions, committees related to self-studies of areas within the institution or the institution as a whole, administrator evaluation committees, athletic department oversight, strategic planning committees, and the board of trustees or committees of the board. Some positions may be elected while most are appointed or voluntary. These venues provide important means for the faculty to have a voice in the future direction of the institution. Also, the nursing faculty need to be part of institutional decisions that affect their educational programs. In addition, participation in governance provides important leadership development opportunities for faculty members, and these experiences are invaluable to nurse educators who aspire to assume a leadership role within the nursing education unit. Yet, while service on committees of the institution are important in the career of a nurse educator, it is also very important to balance one's time appropriately between the teaching, scholarship, and service expectations of one's particular institution and employment agreement.

SUMMARY

- Nurse educators navigate a significant cultural transition when they move from health care delivery to higher education.
- Nursing education programs are located in a wide variety of types of institutions: schools may be focused on nursing or health professions, schools affiliated with a health system, or colleges and universities that offer a variety of degrees in many disciplines.
- Nurse educators need to be aware of the specific heritage and mission of their institution and how the nursing program supports it.
- Nurse educators need to be conversant with accreditation standards to which their program and institution adhere as they continually evaluate program quality and revise or expand program offerings.
- Nurse educators need to understand the terms of their employment agreement in relation to the balance of their total responsibilities for teaching, scholarship, and service; their on-site schedule; clinical practice; and annual contracted service.
- Promotion of a civil environment is associated with increased productivity and retention of student and faculty talent.
- Particular student populations have specific needs, and societal trends or historical events raise awareness of issues to which educational programs need to respond.
- Faculty need to understand the financial health of their academic unit within the context of the institution.
- Nurse educators serve their programs by representing them through faculty self-governance and serving on institutional committees that determine policy and broadly evaluate the organization's function and outcomes.

Practice Test Questions

1. Which statement does *not* accurately describe a type of institution in which academic nursing programs are found?
   A. Research-intensive university
   B. Health sciences school affiliated with a health system
   C. Religious seminary
   D. Proprietary college

2. Which statement describes a recommendation of the Institute of Medicine *Future of Nursing* report of 2010?
   A. All advanced practice nurses be prepared as Doctors of Nursing Practice starting in 2020.
   B. All associate degree programs transition to baccalaureate programs by 2020.
   C. Eighty percent of baccalaureate-prepared nurses earn master's degrees by 2020.
   D. Eighty percent of all nurses be prepared at a baccalaureate or higher-degree level by 2020.

3. The traditional academic role in an institution of higher education is a balance among which components?
   A. Teaching, scholarship, and service
   B. Clinical practice, teaching, and administration
   C. Teaching, evaluation, and service
   D. Teaching, grant writing, and research

4. A nursing professor stated in the professor's medical-surgical nursing class that in a situation of total physical immobility, the professor would not want life-prolonging interventions. A student complained to the department chair that the student's religious values were disparaged by the professor. Which response would be most appropriate for the department chair?
   A. To explore the faculty member's perception of what occurred
   B. To schedule a disciplinary meeting with the faculty member for violating the student's religious freedom
   C. To prohibit nursing faculty from commenting on their personal preferences in health care
   D. To refer the situation to the institution's chief officer for academic affairs

5. Which option describes a major principle behind the promotion of interprofessional education?
   A. It is personally enriching for students to learn in groups of diverse majors.
   B. Nurses will be less likely to use jargon if they experience interprofessional education.
   C. Interprofessional education promotes communication strategies that improve patient safety.
   D. Significant funding for nursing education is available for interprofessional education.

6. In what important way do nursing faculty differ from most other faculty in colleges and universities?
  A. They are not expected to engage in scholarship.
  B. They may be required to engage in clinical practice.
  C. A terminal degree is not valued in their department or school.
  D. Teaching primarily occurs in practice settings.

7. In what important way do nursing programs in colleges and universities differ from nonprofessional programs?
  A. Nursing students are exempted from the institutional core curriculum.
  B. Nursing faculty place little value on interprofessional collaboration.
  C. Nursing faculty place a low priority on international immersion experiences.
  D. Nursing programs are accountable to external discipline-specific accrediting and government regulatory bodies.

8. Awareness of institutional finances is important to nursing faculty for which reason?
  A. Nursing faculty are expected to cultivate donors.
  B. Financial stress increasingly leads to the closure of educational institutions.
  C. Understanding institutional finances helps nursing faculty make better financial decisions.
  D. If faculty understand the budget, they will ask for fewer resources.

9. A nurse educator is considering employment in a private religious institution. The educator is asked to provide a statement relating how faith influences teaching. What is the best response?
  A. Refuse to provide this on the basis of separation of church and state.
  B. Research the religious organization that the school is affiliated with to be sure that this is a comfortable match.
  C. Write a general statement knowing that it will not be given much importance in the hiring decision.
  D. Ask a clergy person from that religious organization to write it for him.

10. A new nurse educator is a member of the Curriculum Committee. Which situation best reflects similarity between clinical and academic cultures?
  A. The committee disagrees with the dean on the value of SAT examinations for admission.
  B. Junior faculty freely disagree with tenured professors on whether or not clinical practica should be graded.
  C. Priority is given to integrating safety and quality principles throughout the nursing curriculum.
  D. The Curriculum Committee determines that new standards from the accrediting body will be implemented with the freshman class that matriculates in two years.

References

Accreditation Commission for Nursing Education. (2019). *ACEN 2017 accreditation manual* (2nd ed.). Retrieved from http://www.acenursing.net/manuals/SC2017.pdf

American Association of Colleges of Nursing. (2019). Holistic admissions. Retrieved from https://www.aacnnursing.org/Diversity-Inclusion/Holistic-Admissions

American Association of Colleges of Nursing. (2017). Nursing faculty shortage. Retrieved from https://www.aacnnursing.org/News-Information/Fact-Sheets/Nursing-Faculty-Shortage

American Association of Colleges of Nursing. (2006). *The essentials of doctoral education for advanced nursing practice.* Retrieved from https://www.aacnnursing.org/Portals/42/Publications/DNPEssentials.pdf

American Association of University Professors. (2006). Professors of practice. Retrieved from https://www.aaup.org/report/professors-practice

American Association of University Professors. (2014). The inclusion in governance of faculty members holding contingent appointments. Retrieved from https://www.aaup.org/report/inclusion-governance-faculty-members-holding-contingent-appointments

Brook, D., Abu-Rish, E., Chiu, C. R., Hammer, D., Wilson, S. Vorivk, L., ... , Zierler, B. (2013). Interprofessional education in team communications: Working together to improve patient safety. *British Medical Journal of Quality and Safety, 22*(5), 414–423. doi: 10.1136/bmjqs-2012-000952

Brown, E. L. (1948). Nursing for the future. New York, NY: Russell Sage Foundation.

Bureau of Labor Statistics. (2018). Occupational outlook handbook: Registered nurses. Retrieved from https://www.bls.gov/ooh/healthcare/registered-nurses.htm

Carnegie Classification of Institutions of Higher Education. (2019). Definitions and methods. Retrieved from http://carnegieclassifications.iu.edu/definitions.php

Chronicle of Higher Education. (2018). The awakening: Women and power in the academy. Retrieved from https://www.chronicle.com/interactives/the-awakening

College Board. (2019). Average published charges 2017–18 and 2018–19. Retrieved from https://trends.collegeboard.org/college-pricing/figures-tables/average-rates-growth-published-charges-decade

Commission on Collegiate Nursing Education. (2018). Standards for accreditation of baccalaureate and graduate nursing education programs. Retrieved from https://www.aacnnursing.org/Portals/42/CCNE/PDF/Standards-Final-2018.pdf

Commission for Nursing Education Accreditation. (2019). Standards of accreditation. Retrieved from http://www.nln.org/accreditation-services/standards-for-accreditation.

Council of Regional Accrediting Commissions. (2019). C-RAC News. Retrieved from https://www.c-rac.org/

Council for the Advancement and Support of Education. (2019). Fundraising Fundamentals, retrieved from https://www.case.org/resources/fundraising-fundamentals

Fang, D., & Bednash, G. D. (2017). Identifying barriers and facilitators to future nursing faculty careers for DNP students. *Journal of Professional Nursing, 33*(1), 56–67.

Filby, M. (2019, January 10). What will trigger furloughs at Wright State? New 'cost savings' policy explained. *Dayton Daily News.* Retrieved from https://www.daytondailynews.com/news/what-will-trigger-furloughs-wright-state-new-cost-savings-policy-explained/ynWEXzLRSpKiu9ttSJ7BOK/

Flaherty, C. (2019). Evening things out. *Inside Higher Ed.* Retrieved from https://www.insidehighered.com/news/2019/01/30/new-research-says-relatively-simple-interventions-are-effective-addressing-faculty

Gardner, L. (2015). Dilemmas from day 1. *Chronicle of Higher Education,* October 18, 2015. Retrieved from https://www.chronicle.com/article/Dilemmas-From-Day-1/233760

Gregory, G. L., & Chapman, C. (2012). *Differentiated instructional strategies: one size doesn't fit all* (3rd ed.). Thousand Oaks, CA: Sage.

Hollis, L. P. (2015). Bully university? The cost of workplace bullying and employee disengagement in American higher education. *SAGE Open.* Retrieved from https://journals.sagepub.com/doi/full/10.1177/2158244015589997

Institute of Medicine. (2010). *The future of nursing: Leading change, advancing health.* Washington, DC: National Academies Press.

Institute of Medicine. (1999). *To err is human: Building a safer health system.* Washington DC: National Academies Press.

International Civil Aviation Organization. (2019). Aircraft engine emissions. Retrieved from https://www.icao.int/environmental-protection/Pages/aircraft-engine-emissions.aspx

Keeling, A. W. (2018). *History of professional nursing in the United States: Toward a culture of health.* New York, NY: Springer.

Lester, J. (2013). Workplace bullying in higher education. New York, NY: Routledge.

Lindsay, T. (2015). More U.S. colleges poised to go bankrupt, according to three new studies. Forbes, November 28. Retrieved from https://www.forbes.com/sites/tomlindsay/2015/11/28/three-new-studies-more-u-s-colleges-poised-to-go-bankrupt/#537b7468af3e

Lippincott Solutions. (2018). Update on future of nursing report—are we there yet? Retrieved from http://lippincottsolutions.lww.com/blog.entry.html/2018/02/13/update_on_futureof-q5jh.html

Makary, M. A., & Daniel, M. (2016). Medical error—the third leading cause of death in the U.S. *British Medical Journal, 353.* doi: https://doi.org/10.1136/bmj.i2139

Marion, L., Douglas, M., Lavin, M., Barr, N., Gazaway, S., Thomas, L., & Bickford, C. (November 18, 2016). Implementing the new ANA Standard 8: Culturally congruent practice. *Online Journal of Issues in Nursing*, 22(1). DOI: 10.3912/OJIN.Vol22No01PPT20

Meleis, A. I. (2018). *Theoretical nursing: Development and progress* (6th ed.). Philadelphia, PA: Wolters Kluwer Health.

Milesky, J. L., Baptiste, D. L., Foronda, C., Dupler, A. E., & Belcher, A. E. (2015). Promoting a culture of civility in nursing education and practice. *Journal of Nursing Education and Practice*, 5(8). Retrieved from: http://www.sciedupress.com/journal/index.php/jnep/article/view/6596/4294

National League for Nursing. (2018). *Certified nurse educator (CNE®) 2018 candidate handbook*. Washington, DC: Author.

National League for Nursing Certification Commission Certification Test Development Committee. (2012).

The scope of practice for academic nurse educators (2012 rev.). New York, NY: National League for Nursing.

National League of Nursing Education. (1937). *Curriculum guide for schools of nursing*. New York, NY: Author.

Perry, A., & Blincoe, S (2015). Bullies and victims in higher education: a mixed-methods approach. *Journal of Bullying and Social Aggression*, 1(1).

QSEN Institute. (2019). About QSEN. Retrieved from http://qsen.org/about-qsen/

Reichman, H. (2018). Free speech and inclusion. *Academe*, 104(3). Retrieved from https://www.aaup.org/article/free-speech-and-inclusion#.XPa2R1NKhp-

Spector, R. E. (2016). *Cultural diversity in health and illness* (9th ed.). Boston: Pearson.

Zemsky, R. (2013). How to build a faculty culture of change. *Chronicle of Higher Education*, September 30, 2013. Retrieved from https://www.chronicle.com/article/How-to-Build-a-Faculty-Culture/141887

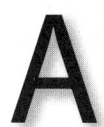

Guide to Educational Learning Theories

Theory	Principles	Application to Learning
Behaviorism	Learning is the result of changes in behavior. Learning is reinforced by response. Stimuli and responses are connected. Prior experience (reinforcements/punishments) determines behaviors. Conditioning determines how individuals respond to a learning situation, as well as the rate at which individuals respond. Theorists: Watson, Skinner, Thorndike	Learning is shaped by others, and students are not held individually responsible for their learning. The teacher and environment hold responsibility for learning. Students are motivated by extrinsic rewards. Use of behavioral course objectives is rooted in behaviorism. Examples of teaching methods: learning contracts and programmed instruction modules.
Cognitivism (Information Processing Theories)	Emphasizes the person's cognitive or thinking processes. Views the learner as more active in the learning process than behaviorism. Learning involves internal processes such as memory, perception, problem solving, reasoning, and concept formation. To acquire information that can be retrieved later, connections to other ideas, prior knowledge, and experience and emotions are necessary. Changes in the learner are an indication of change in cognition. Control for learning is less focused on the environment (behaviorism) and more focused on the learner's mental engagement. Theorists: Brunner, Ausubel, Gagne	Relating incoming information to previously learned information makes it more memorable. The way information is presented to the learner can facilitate and detract from learning. The individual needs to be active in creating a structured network of information (i.e., concept map, comparing ideas, rehearsal, study cards). Examples of teaching methods: group projects, role playing, computerized simulations, teaching foundational facts before higher levels of knowledge.
Social Learning Theory	Hybrid of behaviorist and cognitivist perspectives. Learner and environment are in a reciprocal relationship in which each influences the other. Self-efficacy of one's personal ability and one's sense of self-determination are influential to learning. Modeling or learning through observation is essential. Theorist: Bandura	Learning occurs from passive as well as deliberate observation of behavior. Reflection on the negative consequences of behavior influences limited repetition of the behavior. Teaching methods: self-evaluation of learning, observation of best practices, mastery experiences.

Theory	Principles	Application to Learning
Constructivism	Learning occurs through experience. Learning is actively constructed by the learner and involves actions and reflection of prior experiences to derive meaning. The teaching method is not the determining factor; the active process that the learner uses is key. Learning should include integrating subject matter through application to everyday life. Direct contrast to the passive learning of behaviorism. Learning involves active problem solving, perception, values, and meaning. Theorists: Dewey, Piaget	Students take an active role in learning and construct knowledge out of their own experiences. Peer influences make a difference in learning engagement. It is essential to be able to suspend belief and not be worried about peer pressure to engage in learning. Learners need to motivate from within to have a transformative experience. Examples of teaching methods: making comparisons and associations with previous knowledge, reflective logs, debate.
Humanism	Individuals act with intentionality based on values and needs. Learning is based on human generation of knowledge, meaning, and ultimately expertise through interpersonal and intrapersonal intelligence. The learning goal is to become self-actualized with intrinsic motivation toward accomplishment. The learner is able to adapt prior knowledge to new experiences. Person-centered learning addresses the learner's intellect, social skills, and feelings or intuitions. Theorists: Rogers, Maslow, Freire, Glasser	Acquisition, development, and integration of knowledge occur through strategy, personal interpretation, evaluation, reasoning, and decision-making. The educator's role is to encourage and enable the learner, by providing access to appropriate resources without obtrusive interference. The learning goal is high-order learning of reasoning, abstract analysis, and development of expertise. Teaching methods: classrooms that are student-centered where teachers and students express ideas and perspectives, personal interactions with students that promote positive regard and increase self-esteem.

References

All, A. C., Huycke, L. I., & Fisher, M. J. (2003). Instructional tools for nursing education: Concept maps. *Nursing Education Perspectives, 34,* 311–317.

Bandura, A. (1977). *Social learning theory.* Englewood Cliffs, NJ: Prentice Hall.

Bruner, J. (1964). The course of cognitive growth. *American Psychologst, 19,* 1–15.

Dewey, J. (1910/1997). *How we think.* Mineola, NY: Dover.

Gagne, R. M., Wager, W. W., Golas, K. C., & Keller, J. M. (2005). *Principles of instructional design* (5th ed.). Belmont, CA: Thomas/Wadsworth Publishing.

Hmelo-Silver, C. (2004). Problem-based learning. What and how do students learn? *Educational Psychology Review 16*(3), 235–266.

Kuiper, R., & Pesut, D. (2004). Promoting cognitive and metacognative relective reasoning skills in nursing practice: Self-regulated learning theory. *Journal of Advanced Nursing, 45*(4), 381–391.

Maslow, A. H. (1968). *Toward a psychology of being* (2nd ed.). New York: Van Nostrand.

Rogers, C., & Freiberg, H. J. (1994). *Freedome to learn* (3rd ed.). New York: Charles Merrill.

Slavin, R. E. (2006). *Educational psychology: Theory and practice.* New York: Pearson.

Schunk, D. H. (2012). *Learning theories: An educational perspective* (6th ed.). New York: Pearson.

Utley, R. (2011). *Theory and research for academic nurse educators.* Sudbury, MA: Jonas and Bartlett Publishers.

Answers to Practice Questions

Chapter 1

1. Answer: C

Rationale: Option A: PowerPoint slides are a teacher-focused strategy that provide passive learning. The cognitive domain of application requires the learner to be active in the learning process. Option B: Although students do learn through observing an experienced nurse, the learning does not actively engage the student. The student is not afforded the opportunity to transfer knowledge learned in class and apply it in clinical. Option C: Students are actively discussing the care of the patient in the case study and making clinical decisions demonstrating application of knowledge. Option D: Although students are actively engaged in this learning activity, this game requires recall of knowledge rather than application of knowledge.

2. Answer: B

Rationale: Option A: Case studies encourage active learning, promoting higher-order thinking (Caputi & Frank, 2019). Option B: YouTube videos provide passive learning and may be a great strategy to help students understand concepts/content, but they do not promote higher-order thinking or active learning. Option C: Reflection and journaling promote both active learning and higher-order thinking (Caputi & Frank, 2019). Option D: Students practicing steps of sterile gloving procedure requires active learning but does not promote higher-order thinking.

3. Answer: B

Rationale: Option A: The premise of Adult Learning Theory is that adults are self-directed and problem centered (Candela, 2016). A podcast lecture is passive learning and is not conducive to allowing the learner to solve problems. Option B: Case studies allow the learner to work toward solving a clinical problem. This aligns well with the premise of Adult Learning Theory and can easily be accomplished via an asynchronous online discussion board. Option C: This is an asynchronous online course; thus, role play is not the teaching strategy for this modality. Option D: The use of personal response systems does not allow learners to solve clinical problems. It is also not an appropriate strategy for an asynchronous online course.

4. Answer: C

Rationale: Option A: This statement provides a clear instruction on what to review; however, the heart "pumping" blood is jargon. Stating that the heart circulates blood would be more effective for a student who is an English language learner. Option B: "Crit" is medical jargon. The ANE should state the exact word for clarity. Option C: This statement is very clear, concise, and avoids the use of abbreviations. Option D: The term "weed" is jargon. The ANE should state the exact term: "marijuana."

5. Answer: D

Rationale: Option A: This provides only written information, which is a good strategy for visual learners. However, this will be challenging for auditory and kinesthetic learners (Rundle & Dunn, 2008) or students who are English language learners (Billings, 2015). Option B: This provides only written information, which is a good strategy for visual learners. However, this will be challenging for auditory and kinesthetic learners (Rundle & Dunn, 2008) or students who are English language learners (Billings, 2015). Option C: Students always welcome examples of assignments. However, this provides only written information, which is a good strategy for visual learners and will be challenging for auditory and kinesthetic learners (Rundle & Dunn, 2008) or students who are English language learners (Billings, 2015). Option D: This will present the instructions both verbally and in writing, which meets the needs of diverse learning styles and students who are English language learners.

6. Answer: A

Rationale: Option A: Guided imagery is a strategy that faculty can use to practice self-awareness to better understand themselves and their learners (Rasheed,

Younas, & Sundus, 2018). "Self-reflection and self-awareness are at the core of co-creating environments for respect and civility" (NLN, 2018b, p. 4). Option B: Although this is a good strategy, as the nurse faculty is practicing communication, it does not allow the faculty to practice self-awareness on the thoughts/feelings of the faculty and student, which are needed for respect and civility. Option C: Although the list will ensure that all points are addressed in the evaluation, it does not necessarily promote reflections on the thoughts/feelings of the faculty and student, which are needed for respect and civility. Option D: Although it is important to maintain student privacy, it does not consider the thoughts/feelings of faculty and student, which ensure respect and civility.

7. Answer: D

Rationale: Option A: Although the student comment is positive, the comment reflects faculty practice of passive learning. The PowerPoint slides offered so much information that the student did not even need to take notes during faculty lecture. Option B: This student offers great comments on the faculty's attributes, which can assist in facilitating learning. The faculty's use of technology also facilitates learning, but the comment does not indicate that the student is actively engaged in learning. Option C: This comment brings to light the faculty's attributes in creating a positive learning environment, but there is no mention of active learning by students. Option D: This comment demonstrates that the faculty member has created a positive, engaging learning environment and that students are active in the learning process with concept mapping.

8. Answer: B

Rationale: Option A: Using YouTube videos and photos with PowerPoint meets the technology preferences of millennials (Popkess & Frey, 2016). However, this strategy does not allow learners to make decisions. Option B: Using personal response systems meets the technology preferences of millennials (Popkess & Frey, 2016). Furthermore using NCLEX-style questions engages higher-level thinking and decision-making (Efstathiou & Bailey, 2012; Mareno et al., 2010; Revell & McCurry, 2010). Option C: Socratic questioning engages higher-level learning and clinical judgment (Carvalho et al., 2017; Paul & Elder, 2013; Phillips, 2016). However, this strategy might not completely appeal to the millennial learner. Option D: Having students write practice NCLEX-style questions engages higher-level learning and clinical judgment (Paul & Elder, 2013;

Carvalho et al., 2017; Phillips, 2016). However, this strategy might not completely appeal to the millennial learner.

9. Answer: A

Rationale: Option A: This option demonstrates flexibility of the nurse educator to reasonably work with the student. Option B: This option demonstrates flexibility of the nurse educator only and is not compassionate since the student will most likely be at the height of grief the day before the funeral. Option C: This option does not demonstrate any caring behaviors. Option D: This option demonstrates compassion only and does not address the student's worry about missing the exam.

10. Answer: B

Rationale: Option A: Socratic questioning asks questions to analyze individual thinking (Phillips, 2016). Although it occurs in a group setting, it does not offer the opportunity to work as a team. Option B: Collaborative testing allows for critical thinking and team-based learning (Wiggs, 2010). Option C: Case studies allow for problem solving in a safe environment and may be assigned as an individual assignment or a group assignment (Phillips, 2016). For this activity to promote team function, it must be assigned as a group. This option does not identify the case study as being assigned as group work. Option D: Having students create algorithms is active learning and assists in teaching problem-solving techniques or teaching complex procedures (Phillips, 2016). However, this strategy does not have students working in teams.

11. Answer: C

Rationale: Option A: This option may be uncivil as it calls attention to the students' poor behaviors in front of their peers. It would be appropriate for the nurse educator to have a private conversation with these students. Option B: Although this behavior might not be disturbing the other students, this option allows these students to remain unengaged, which may be counterproductive to achieving learning outcomes. Option C: This option actively engages the students in the class without bringing attention to their disengagement. It also brings the use of technology into the classroom. Option D: This option may be uncivil, as it calls attention to the students' poor behaviors in front of their peers. It would be appropriate for the nurse educator to have a private conversation with these students.

12. Answer: D

Rationale: Option A: This option demonstrates that the nurse educator is diving into the literature to find teaching strategies that support a positive learning environment. Positive learning environments facilitate learning, as discussed in this chapter. Option B: This option shows that the nurse educator is taking into account the student preferences but also the evidence behind the flipped classroom along with support of improved test scores. Option C: This option shows that the nurse educator is diving into the literature to find evidence-based online teaching strategies for student engagement. Option D: This option demonstrates the importance of student feedback as evidence, but the educator is not taking into account the poor outcomes of passive learning. The plan is to change based only on student preferences. This option requires further mentoring.

13. Answer: A

Rationale: Option A: A premise of Social Cognitive Theory is that students learn through observation of others (Candela, 2016). Option B: Although this is an active learning strategy, it does not include any premise of Social Cognitive Theory. There is no observation or learning with others. Option C: Although this is an active learning strategy, it does not include any premise of Social Cognitive Theory. There is no observation or learning with others. Option D: There is no observation or learning with others.

14. Answer: B

Rationale: Option A: This nurse educator is addressing a generational need but the policy of only using eBooks is not inclusive of other students who do not favor technology. Option B: Learner needs include the individual prerequisite knowledge, skills, and attitudes that learners have prior to starting the nursing programs. This response demonstrates that the nurse educator assesses previous health experience when making group activity assignments. Option C: In this option, the nurse educator is considering the diverse learning styles of students but not learner needs. Option D: This option demonstrates that the nurse educator is using an active learning strategy in lecture but does not consider individual learner needs.

15. Answer: C

Rationale: Option A: Although this strategy promotes collaboration with the staff nurse, it does not promote active learning. Option B: This strategy is passive learning and is not the best for learning.

Option C: This response has the student actively engaged in problem solving in the clinical setting and promotes self-directed learning. Reporting the findings in post-conference promotes student empowerment. Option D: Although this strategy has the student actively collaborating and learning with the clinical instructor, it does not promote the additional benefit of student empowerment.

16. Answer: B

Rationale: Option A: Although it is good practice to have an orientation to the unit, the nurse educator needs to collaborate with the clinical site for a day/time that works for the site. Option B: The nurse educator needs to communicate the clinical objectives with the unit manager so that the clinical site is aware of the learning outcomes. Option C: Although this strategy may work at some clinical sites, it will not work at all clinical sites. This practice should be done only after collaborating with the clinical site. Option D: The nurse educator should work with the unit manager when assigning patients since the nurse educator best knows the students' learning needs.

17. Answer: A

Rationale: Option A: The baby boomer generation was taught with the teacher-centered approach. To meet the needs of this generation, the nurse educator should integrate more lecture in class (Popkess & Frey, 2016). Option B: Baby boomers did not grow up with technology; therefore, they may struggle more if this technology is added in the class. Option C: Baby boomers did not grow up with technology; therefore, they may struggle more if this technology is added as homework. Option D: Although concept mapping is an active learning activity that needs to be included in the teaching plan, the baby boomer generation prefers teacher-centered lecture (Popkess & Frey, 2016).

18. Answer: A

Rationale: Option A: Socratic questioning is an active learning strategy that promotes critical thinking (Phillips, 2016). Option B: Lecture is a passive learning strategy that is teacher focused and does not promote critical thinking. Option C: Although a one-minute paper is an active learning strategy, it does not give enough time for students to think critically and students are focused only on disease complications. They are not correlating physiological changes with both clinical manifestations and complications. Option D: Showing a movie is a passive learning strategy that does not promote critical thinking.

19. Answer: D

Rationale: Option A: Informing students of the objectives before any learning activity promotes a positive learning environment. This does not require further guidance. Option B: Reviewing student expectations of appropriate behaviors for simulation will create a civil and positive learning environment. This does not require further guidance. Option C: Requesting student volunteers demonstrates the faculty member's willingness to allow students to make decisions related to the learning activity, promoting a positive learning environment. Option D: Although it is important to have students learn from their mistakes, the students need to recognize their errors rather than have them highlighted and be the focus of debriefing. The debriefing session needs to be student focused and respectful. Highlighting errors is not respectful, can be perceived as judgmental by students, and requires further guidance.

20. Answer: C

Rationale: Option A: Although this a great strategy for building a relationship between the clinical agency and students, it does not encourage the students to learn through role modeling. Option B: Although the students may be motivated to learn when they know the skills that they are able to perform, it does not encourage learning through role modeling. Option C: By sharing credentials and previous history of clinical experiences, the ANE is communicating competence with the students. According to Reader et al. (2017), nursing students perceive faculty as a positive role model when they demonstrate clinical competence. Furthermore, when faculty show enjoyment and interest in the subject matter, they are better able to motivate and inspire students (Lerret & Frenn, 2011; Sedden & Clark, 2016). Option D: Although providing written documentation of clinical objectives and expectations is important to creating a positive learning environment, it may not effectively motivate students. Furthermore, it does not encourage the students to learn through role modeling.

Chapter 2

1. Answer: D

Rationale: Options A and B are information-based, consistent with prescriptive advising. Option C attends to broader holistic development, consistent with developmental advising. Option D attempts to help mitigate a problem, consistent with intrusive advising.

2. Answer: C

Rationale: In addition to expected language barriers, EAL students often experience additional challenges when learning medical terminology and medical axioms. Providing a reference sheet may help in their understanding of commonly used health care language. Options A, B, and D are not recommended, as the instructor would not be responsible for providing translator services, students pick up a new language quicker when teamed with others who speak it, and class work typically takes longer for EAL students.

3. Answer: A

Rationale: Option A: Professional identity formation is a personal process that requires acceptance of professional values as demonstrated by one's personal and professional behaviors. Options B and C suggest that the process is external to the nurse, while Option D suggests professional identity is a static trait.

4. Answer: D

Rationale: Option D: Private discussion with the student soon after the incident ensures that the events will be fresh in the minds of both instructor and student while preventing embarrassment and building additional trust. Options A, B, and C all jeopardize accurate memory or erode the trusting relationship.

5. Answer: A

Rationale: Option A represents the period of exploration associated with emerging adulthood. Option B is a lower-level developmental task consistent with adolescence. Options C and D are consisted with higher-level developmental tasks.

6. Answer: A

Rationale: Option A: Active experimentation involves taking previously learned knowledge and applying it in new situations. Options B, C, and D are incorrect because they involve other Kolb stages of learning.

7. Answer: C

Rationale: Option C: Divergers learn by feeling and watching; a film followed by reflection would likely be most meaningful to them. Options A, B, and D are more appropriate for other learning styles.

8. Answer: A

Rationale: Option A: Convergers learn by thinking and doing, such as in hands-on experimentation and practical problem-solving. Options B,

C, and D are more appropriate for other learning styles.

9. Answer: A

Rationale: Option A: Adult learners expand on their previous experiences and learning when learning new material. Options B, C, and D are not conducive to adult learning. It is important for the nurse educator to collaborate with adult learners in identifying learning needs and developing learning experiences to meet those needs. In general, adult learners tend to be more self-directed and require less structure to meet learning outcomes.

10. Answer: A

Rationale: Option A: In a concept map, the student expresses the concept and its relationship to other elements in a visual format. Using maps, the student thinks critically, synthesizes and organizes content, and demonstrates relationships. Option B: Algorithms are maps that break down decision-making issues into step-by-step procedures that lead to yes or no answers or varying action choices. They do not demonstrate relationships but are best used to teach the steps of a complex procedure. Option C: The one-minute paper is best used to assess the comprehension of major course concepts but would lack the depth to analyze the complexity of an ill-structured case study. Option D: Simulation is best to evaluate skills in a more authentic environment but would not meet this objective.

11. Answer: D

Rationale: Option D is correct as it requires knowledge synthesis to create a plan of care that did not previously exist. Options A, B, and C represent lower levels of cognitive learning.

12. Answer: C

Rationale: Option C: To best master a skill (the psychomotor domain) the student should practice consistently and over time. Through consistent repetition, the more experienced nurse is able to internalize skills so that the performance becomes natural and precise. An instructor should be student friendly and foster development. With a complex skill, the instructor should allow time for remediation and coach the student until proficient in this skill. The other strategies (Options B and D, paper and reflection in a journal or orally, respectively) would not be appropriate for a manual skill. Option A is unacceptable; the student must be provided due process, which involves helping to remediate the student and then reevaluating.

13. Answer: D

Rationale: Option D: Interaction between teachers and students is the most important factor in engaging students with the material to be studied and facilitating their learning. The other options do not directly encourage faculty-student interactions.

14. Answer: C

Rationale: Option C: The affective domain of learning reflects the student's growth in feelings or emotional areas. The student demonstrates belief in the value of an individual. This ranges from simple acceptance to the more complex state of commitment. The other options do not foster the student's growth in the affective domain.

15. Answer: D

Rationale: Option D: Difficulties experienced by EAL students are frequently the result of language issues. Research suggests that pairing EAL students with native English speakers who can coach them in proper use and understanding of English helps improve overall language proficiency. Options A, B, and C do not put the EAL student into discussions with native English speakers.

16. Answer: A

Rationale: Option A: How students take in knowledge and make sense of it is key to experiential learning, which Kolb considers a requirement for adaptation. Thus, in order to learn, new information is constantly compared to what is known from previous experience. Ultimately, either the previous experiences or the new knowledge is seen in a new light, as the learner adapts beliefs, values, and understanding. Options B, C, and D are not reflective of experiential learning theory.

17. Answer: D

Rationale: While Options A, B, and C are all important, the nurse educator ultimately has responsibility for patient safety (Option D). Evidence is mounting suggesting that disruptive behavior and incivility in the workplace jeopardize patient safety. Thus, it is increasingly essential that students and new graduates display appropriate relational skills.

18. Answer B

Rationale: Option B is correct because the student is able to reflect on study and other habits that have an impact on student performance. Options A, C, and D all involve relatively concrete tasks.

19. Answer: B

Rationale: Option B is correct. Option A: Students must self-disclose disabilities and formally request accommodation under the ADA. Option C: Reasonable accommodations must be offered and are considered within the context of a program's resources. Option D: Although accommodations may include adjusting clinical experiences or modifying examinations, ultimately the student must successfully achieve the established program objectives.

20. Answer: C

Rationale: Option C is correct because it requires the student to value the impact of sociocultural influences. Options A and D represent the cognitive domain, while Option B is aligned with the psychomotor domain.

Chapter 3

1. Answer: A

Rationale: Faculty should consider all data when implementing a standardized test policy. Options B and C are not supported by data, and Option D does not accurately reflect fair testing policies.

2. Answer: D

Rationale: Formative assessment occurs during the assessment period and supports modification of instruction. Options A, B, and C are not related.

3. Answer: C

Rationale: Guiding questions in summative evaluation include "Were behavioral objectives of the clinical course met?" and "Did the individual(s) learn?" Options A and B assess learning during one certain time and are not summative, and Option D is program evaluation.

4. Answer: B

Rationale: Options A, C, and D are examples of norm-referenced interpretation. Criterion-referenced interpretation of data is used typically in competency-based models to achieve competence in, or mastery of, specified learning outcomes.

5. Answer: A

Rationale: A comprehensive portfolio can best demonstrate overall achievement of program learning outcomes. While Option B may address specific competencies, it is unlikely to reflect all learning outcomes. Options C and D are both student reflections, which may not reflect program outcomes.

6. Answer: C

Rationale: A short-answer quiz addresses knowledge-level understanding, while Option A asks students to "demonstrate," which would better address an objective related to *demonstrate*. An essay is better for higher-level verbs, such as *apply* or *analyze*, and creating a poster on how to change a dressing may not demonstrate "understand concepts."

7. Answer: D

Rationale: Option D is the only answer that permits students to "demonstrate" the process. Options A, B, and C are all cognitive measures but do not meet the psychomotor technique of demonstration.

8. Answer: A

Rationale: A reflective journal is most effective at capturing emotions, feelings, and values. The cognitive and psychomotor domains are not well reflected in a journal. Option C is not a domain.

9. Answer: B

Rationale: Prioritization demonstrates application of all parts of the nursing process, whereas Options A, C, and D each focus on only one area of the nursing process.

10. Answer: D

Rationale: This is a knowledge level objective and asks students to recall definitions. Options A, B, and C would not meet the objective of "define terms."

11. Answer: C

Rationale: Prioritizing requires higher-level application of knowledge to a situation. Options A, B, and D are knowledge- and comprehension-level questions that do not ask for application of knowledge.

12. Answer: A

Rationale: A final exam is designed to assess comprehension of course concepts. Options B and D reflect clinical applications, and Option C is a self-reflection.

13. Answer: C

Rationale: If there are several faculty members teaching a course and responsible for a group of students in that course, interrater reliability must be established to maintain consistency, eliminate bias, and ensure fairness for all students in the class. Options A and B are not feasible, and Option D does not address laboratory and clinical evaluation.

14. Answer: D

Rationale: Both test answer options have a PBI of greater than 0.20, indicating discrimination between low-scoring and high-scoring students. For Option A, reliability is high; Option B indicates that the higher-scoring students answered the item correctly. For Option C, the acceptable range for difficulty is generally between 70 percent and 80 percent, although variation can occur.

15. Answer: A

Rationale: The difficulty value (p value) indicates the percent of students who selected the correct answer. Option B is incorrect because a negative PBI indicates that low-scoring students selected this answer more than high-scoring students. Option C is incorrect as more high-scoring students selected this answer. Option D is incorrect as the overall PBI of 0.10 does not discriminate at greater than 0.20, the desired minimum.

16. Answer: D

Rationale: A p value of less than .70 indicates more difficult items. A low KR-20 shows poor reliability and should be greater than 0.60. The p value and KR-20 are not related to discriminating between low- and high-scoring students.

17. Answer: D

Rationale: The purpose of item analysis is to look for items that are too difficult, too easy, or had multiple correct answers. Options A, B, and C are not valid purposes of an item analysis.

18. Answer: C

Rationale: The p value of 1.00 means that no students selected the distractors. Option A may be true but cannot be assumed from the results. For Option B, students had the correct answer. In Option D, the item was too easy, not too difficult.

19. Answer A

Rationale: The response is asking the student to demonstrate understanding of respiratory precautions by selecting which option would require respiratory precautions. Options B, C, and D require higher-level thinking in the Bloom's taxonomy range.

20. Answer: C

Rationale: Option A is understanding, and Options B and D are applying.

Chapter 4

1. Answer: B

Rationale: Option B takes into consideration the level of the nursing student in the program. The competency must reflect that level of functioning. A student in the last semester should be engaging in the behavior in Option B. Option A refers to "basic plans of care." Option C does not engage the student in the higher-level activity of delegating. Option D refers to patients with "common" medical-surgical problems. By the last semester, students should be caring for complex patients.

2. Answer: A

Rationale: Option A: The first step in developing a curriculum is to determine the desired characteristics of the new graduates. Option B: The curriculum is old; thus, the theoretical framework for that curriculum is outdated. Options C and D are tasks that will be completed but come later in the curriculum revision process.

3. Answer: D

Rationale: Option D: Course content must build on that of prerequisite nursing courses. Option A is incorrect because the two nursing programs may be structured differently. Option B is incorrect because the textbook is a reference but not the guide to the curriculum; not all information in the textbook may be important information to be taught. Option C is incorrect because although faculty are expert nurses, personal opinion may guide decisions, leading to content that is taught for the wrong reasons.

4. Answer: B

Rationale: Option B is correct because it provides the overall purpose of the program assessment plan. Options A, C, and D are addressed in an assessment plan, but they do not represent the overall purpose of a program assessment plan.

5. Answer: A

Rationale: Option A is correct because it provides an open-ended question that specifically addresses what nurses do in the current health care environment. This is important information for developing a current curriculum. Option B might yield institution-specific information that may not be generalized for other institutions. Option C elicits a yes/no answer that does not provide useful information. Option D is not related to the purpose of the program.

6. Answer: A, C, E

Rationale: Options A, C, and E are all reliable sources of credible, professional information. Option B is incorrect because it addresses the wrong level of nursing. Option D is incorrect because *Wikipedia* is not a professional site.

7. Answer: D

Rationale: Option D: It is best to have a program-wide approach for selecting content for all nursing courses. Option A: Selection of content should be based on a program policy, not on an individual faculty member's decision. Option B: It is necessary to teach all content listed on the NCLEX test plan in a prelicensure program; however, other content not on the NCLEX is important to teach as well. Option C: Faculty typically have no information about how standardized testing companies select specific content to include on their exams. Faculty own the curriculum and as such should make the curriculum decision, not an outside testing company.

8. Answer: B

Rationale: Option B: Research has demonstrated that using a framework to teach clinical judgment across the curriculum has the best results. Option A: There is no evidence that with increased exposure nursing students become better thinkers in nursing. Option C: There is no evidence that current strategies for teaching thinking are effective. Option D: Although nursing students are adults and may know how to think, they do not know how to think in nursing; therefore, having a systematic, planned approach for teaching thinking is critical.

9. Answer: B

Rationale: Option B: Technology should be used for a specific educational purpose. Options A and D do not include an educational purpose. Option C is incorrect because many virtual simulations can deliver a realistic experience, especially for patient experiences that are not available.

10. Answer: A

Rationale: Option A: Lesson plans lay out the connections among the various components of the curriculum, demonstrating internal consistency. Option B: Test blueprints provide information only about how each test item is connected to various aspects of the curriculum. Option C: A systematic plan of evaluation is used to evaluate all aspects of a nursing program, not just the curriculum. Option D: The model used to deliver the curriculum content provides information about how content is organized for delivery, such as the traditional body systems model or the concept-based curriculum. It does not provide information that supports evidence of internal consistency.

Chapter 5

1. Answer: B

Rationale: Making students aware of their personal responsibilities related to honesty and integrity within a course, as outlined in the course syllabus, provides students guidance. Option B is a priority. Options A, C, and D are not.

2. Answer: D

Rationale: Commitments to building a career and to one's personal life and responsibilities typically need to be balanced. Option D suggests the need for mentoring toward better balance. Finding overlap in work and scholarly products and working with teams are often ways to help with this balance. Options A, C, and D provide this guidance. A, B, & C

3. Answer: C

Rationale: Legal/ethical issues are diverse. Option C would be a concern since it violates Health Insurance Portability and Accountability Act guidelines. Knowing basic guides helps faculty focus their best response. Options A, B, and D provide that direction.

4. Answer: C

Rationale: Proactive strategies such as orientation to handbooks and policies that help students avoid intentional plagiarism are best. Option C indicates a student concern. Options A, B, and D provide proactive strategies.

5. Answer: B

Rationale: Multiple and diverse strategies for gaining feedback are considered best practices in promoting honest assessment and ongoing quality improvement. Option B indicates a concern. Options A, C, and D provide direction.

6. Answer: D

Rationale: Seeking a good job/career fit includes seeking a mesh between career interests and organizational missions. Option D is a concern, as it does not indicate a match with the community college mission. Options A, B, C provide this direction in clarifying interests.

7. Answer: A

Rationale: Building one's CV helps document career progression. Option A indicates a concern. Options B, C, and D provide direction.

8. Answer: B

Rationale: Processes for gaining an academic promotion are very specific and typically adhere to a strict calendar and process. Option B indicates a concern. Options A, C, and D provide direction.

9. Answer: A

Rationale: Professional organizations provide a conduit to current events and evidence-based approaches in a specialty or profession. Option A indicates a concern. Options B, C, and D provide direction.

10. Answer: C

Rationale: New faculty "typically" need guidance in new academic roles. This will include orientation not only to the specific nursing program but also the larger academic organization and associated clinical agencies. Option C indicates a concern, as new faculty may not be aware of the impact of the larger organization. Options A, B, and D provide direction.

11. Answer: B

Rationale: Building a scholarly portfolio requires planning, efficiency, and focus. This is best met when there is a match with organization, mentor, and faculty interests and needs. Option B indicates a concern, as it leaves faculty out of the planning process. Options A, C, and D provide direction.

12. Answer: B

Rationale: Being aware of legal resources and policies provides guidance and is important to the faculty role. Option B is a concern since the student should be aware of his status and potential for failing. Options A, C, and D provide direction.

Chapter 6

1. Answer: C

Rationale: Option A: This is incorrect because it is managers who tend to focus on task accomplishment and leaders who have a long-term perspective. Option B: This is incorrect because it is managers whose power comes from their "official" role in the organization and the authority to reward or punish others; leaders' power comes from what they know, their credibility, and the

trustworthy relationships that they build. Option C: This is correct. According to Grossman & Valiga (2017) and Zaleznik (1981), leaders focus on long-term goals, articulate goals that arise from their passion for excellence, collaborate with followers, and have power because of what they know. In contrast, managers focus on task accomplishment, articulate goals that are formulated by the organization, direct subordinates in their work, and have power because of their formal position of authority in the organization. Option D: This is incorrect because leaders do not have "subordinates," nor do they typically "direct" those with whom they are collaborating to realize a vision.

2. Answer: B

Rationale: Option A: This is incorrect because surveying faculty about the need for change is not necessarily an indication of an individual's cultural sensitivity. Option B: This is correct. By acknowledging that each individual who will participate in the change process is unique and likely to react to and engage with the process in different ways because of that uniqueness, the nursing education leader role models cultural sensitivity. Option C: This is incorrect. While asking representatives from various subgroups to review a proposal for change might suggest a desire to obtain the perspectives of various groups, those subgroups may not necessarily have any relation to cultural diversity. Option D: This is incorrect because attending lectures on diversity, while informative, is not necessarily an indication of an individual's cultural sensitivity.

3. Answer: B

Rationale: Option A: This is incorrect because merely reviewing evaluations of a curriculum development presentation may provide information about the extent to which the presentation helped faculty understand curriculum design, but it does not necessarily give any indication of their readiness to undertake a major curriculum change. Option B: This is correct. Readiness for change can best be evaluated by gaining an understanding of the extent and nature of change recently experienced by the group as well as understanding the degree to which administration supports a proposed change. If members of a group have been involved in extensive change over a lengthy period of time, if past experiences with change have been negative, or if individuals perceive that the administration is not supportive of a proposed change—and may, indeed, say that the change cannot be implemented—their willingness to participate in yet another major change is likely to be quite limited. Option C: This is incorrect because while comments made at a meeting may be a clue to the individual attempting to lead the curriculum change that faculty are or are not aligned with the goals of the change, such information is not indicative of their readiness for transformative change in the curriculum. Option D: This is incorrect because learning about the nursing practice experiences of faculty is not helpful in determining their readiness to engage in curriculum revision work.

4. Answer: C

Rationale: Option A: This is incorrect. While it might be important to consider workload implications, when implementing educational change, attention to such details is relevant only after the vision of a preferred future is articulated, as was done by this nursing education leader. Option B: This is incorrect. While it might be important to consider relationships with clinical partners when implementing educational change, attention to such details is relevant only after the vision of a preferred future is articulated, as was done by this nursing education leader. Option C: This is correct. A nursing education leader can demonstrate one's passion for new ideas and articulate a vision of a more effective, engaging, meaningful educational experience for students by explicating a radically different approach to course design and implementation. Such a vision is needed to help colleagues consider and, indeed, move to create a better program. When such a vision evolves from a synthesis of research findings and recommendations from experts in the field, one can be confident that it defines a preferred future—one that is desirable and is an improvement over what now exists. Option D: This is incorrect. While it might be important to consider program evaluation standards when implementing educational change, attention to such details is relevant only after the vision of a preferred future is articulated, as was done by this nursing education leader.

5. Answer: A

Rationale: Option A: This is correct. Effective leaders help others see a better way to do things and motivate those individuals to join in making those things happen. In other words, they clearly articulate a vision and motivate others to help realize it. Option B: This is incorrect because change and innovation will not necessarily occur due to the fact that the individual advocating for it holds a position of authority in an organization or is tenured. Although such individuals may have significant influence in an organization, they do not

provide any assurance that others in the organization will be willing to invest the time and energy needed to create change and implement innovative approaches to teaching, assessment, curriculum design, new faculty orientation, and so on. Option C: This is incorrect because change and innovation will not necessarily occur due to the fact that the individual advocating for it holds the rank of professor or chairs a committee. Although such individuals may have a significant influence in an organization, they do not provide any assurance that others in the organization will be willing to invest the time and energy needed to create change and implement innovative approaches to teaching, assessment, curriculum design, new faculty orientation, and so on. Option D: This is incorrect because change and innovation will not necessarily occur due to the fact that the individual advocating for it outlines tasks to be done and timelines to be achieved. Although such activities may be helpful, they do not provide any assurance that others in the organization will be willing to invest the time and energy needed to create change and implement innovative approaches to teaching, assessment, curriculum design, new faculty orientation, and so on.

6. Answer: D

Rationale: Option A: This is incorrect. Keeping focused on the present and ensuring that policies are implemented as prescribed typically is the responsibility of a manager or administrator and is not usually expected of followers. Option B: This is incorrect. While effective followers do challenge new ideas, they are not interested in maintaining the status quo but, instead, strive to invest efforts to help the leader achieve the expressed vision about which they are excited. Option C: This is incorrect. While effective followers do listen to discussions about a proposed initiative, they do not accept tasks blindly but, instead, offer ideas about how to get the work done. Option D: This is correct. Effective followers think critically, challenge ideas, question the status quo, do not follow blindly, are not stuck in the present, and do more than merely listen. They participate actively and collaborate with the leader to make things happen.

7. Answer: C

Rationale: Option A: This is incorrect. While an individual faculty member may be tasked with leading strategic planning efforts for the school and other faculty often are asked to provide input throughout the process, it typically is the dean/chair/director who assumes that responsibility.

Option B: This is incorrect. While faculty may be asked to provide input as the school's budget is being developed, responsibility for making final decisions about the budget and strategic plan and overseeing their implementation rests with the individual in the designated position of authority. Option C: This is correct. Any faculty member (including the dean/chair) who is providing leadership within the school may help members of the faculty engage in evidence-based teaching practices. Indeed, providing such help may be a strategy implemented by the nursing education leader to facilitate change on a larger scale. Option D: This is incorrect. Typically, it is the dean/chair/director who acts as the spokesperson for the school within the parent institution, though this may be delegated to individual faculty in certain circumstances. When such a role is delegated, however, the representing faculty member is expected to convey the perspectives of the dean/director.

8. Answer: A

Rationale: Option A: This is correct. The nurse educator who accepts an invitation or nomination to have one's name placed on a ballot for election to office in a national organization is exhibiting leadership and a desire to influence the future directions of that organization. Even if the individual is not elected to office, the fact that educator took the risk, was viewed as someone with ideas/perspectives to offer that could benefit the organization, and expressed a willingness to work in a larger forum to create change all suggest qualities of a leader. Option B: This is incorrect. While maintaining a practice is laudable, it is not necessarily an indication of leadership or a willingness to facilitate change. Option C: This is incorrect because leaders strive for excellence and do not settle for mediocrity or the status quo; therefore, advocating to keep things as they are simply because there are no major negative outcomes of the existing curriculum is not characteristic of a leader or change agent. Option D: This is incorrect. Talking with students about the importance of scholarly work and professional involvement is valuable, but it does not necessarily mean that the faculty member actually takes on such responsibilities.

9. Answer: D

Rationale: Option A: This is incorrect. Serving as chair of a committee within the school may reflect leadership within that limited community but does little to enhance the visibility of nursing at the institutional level. Option B: This is incorrect. Volunteering at a local clinic enhances the visibility of nursing, but it is within the community rather than

in the parent institution. Option C: This is incorrect. Merely attending any kind of meeting does not indicate leadership and, while it is likely to be noted that "nursing has a representative" at the faculty senate meeting, lack of active involvement in those meetings will not serve to enhance the visibility of nursing within the institution. Option D: This is correct. Coordinating a health fair for members of the institutional community best demonstrates leadership, clearly reflects the professional expertise of nurses, and serves to enhance the visibility of nursing within and its contributions to the parent institution.

10. Answer: B

Rationale: Option A: This is incorrect. There is no separate data-gathering stage in Lewin's theory, though relevant data will need to be gathered during the unfreezing stage. Option B: This is correct. Lewin's change theory outlines three stages: unfreezing, moving, and refreezing. In the first stage, participants explore the need for change, discuss the implications of the change, begin to appreciate the effort that will be involved to implement and sustain the change, and realize how they will need to change once the new approach is in place. All of this, understandably, makes many participants anxious and fearful. As a result, they may resist efforts to move toward making changes. Option C: This is incorrect. While some members of the group may try to sabotage or undermine the change once it has been implemented and is being integrated into "the new normal," these are not concerns facing the leader at the beginning of the change process. Option D: This is incorrect. While financial support may be lacking as the change is being put into place, this is not a primary concern facing the leader at the beginning of the change process.

Chapter 7

1. Answer: A

Rationale: Option A: Scholarship of discovery entails research; thus, this is correct. Option B: Scholarship of discovery entails research; thus, this is not correct. Option C: Scholarship of discovery entails research; thus, this is not correct. Option D: Scholarship of discovery entails research; thus, this is not correct.

2. Answer: D

Rationale: Option A: Scholarship of discovery entails research; thus, this is not correct. Option B: Scholarship of discovery entails research; thus, this is not correct. Option C: Scholarship of discovery entails research; thus, this is not correct. Option D: Scholarship of discovery entails research; thus, this is correct.

3. Answer: C

Rationale: Option A: Service to the institution would be part of the scholarship of application, not teaching. Option B: Ethnocentric learning experiences would be poor practice, not the scholarship of teaching. Option C: Sharing results of a teaching experience constitutes the scholarship of teaching; thus, this is correct. Option D: Practicing as a nurse could be scholarship of application if it was planned, evaluated by those receiving the service, and broadened the nurse educator's expertise, but it is not an example of the scholarship of teaching.

4. Answer: A

Rationale: Option A: Service related to one's area of expertise is characteristic of the Scholarship of Application; thus, this is correct. Option B: Service related to one's area of expertise is characteristic of the Scholarship of Application, not Scholarship of Integration. Option C: Service related to one's area of expertise is characteristic of the Scholarship of Application, not Scholarship of Discovery. Option D: Service related to one's area of expertise is characteristic of the Scholarship of Application, not Scholarship of Teaching.

5. Answer: D

Rationale: Option A: Service related to one's area of expertise is characteristic of the Scholarship of Application, but it needs to include evaluations of the work *by those served* (though peer evaluations and publications address other areas of scholarship). Option B: Service related to one's area of expertise (not any type of service) is characteristic of the Scholarship of Application. Option C: Providing a health fair would only be Scholarship of Application if one was needed as determined by members of the community, rather than to facilitate student interaction. Option D: Service that broadens the nurse educator's understanding of the field is characteristic of the Scholarship of Application; thus, this is correct.

6. Answer: B

Rationale: Option A: An educational innovation would need to be based on evidence; "innovations" that are teaching as one was taught would not be an example of evidence-based teaching. Option B: This is the best answer, since the literature is consulted based on an established process

that includes attention to cost, nurse educator expertise, and student perspectives. Option C: Evidence-based teaching may not be the way a course has always been taught, though that information may be helpful in planning. Option D: Student perspectives are some of the evidence to be considered in evidence-based teaching.

7. Answer: D

Rationale: Option A: Syllabi may be helpful, but the expertise needs to be evaluated; thus, this is not the best answer. Option B: Attending programs may be helpful, but it does not demonstrate sharing of teaching expertise. Option C: Course work may be helpful, but it does not demonstrate sharing of teaching expertise. Option D: This is the best answer, since it provides an evaluated sharing of expertise.

8. Answer: A

Rationale: Option A: This is the best answer since protecting client autonomy is included in professional nursing ethical codes. Option B: Providing feedback about professional ethics does not violate the student's right to free speech. Option C: It would be inappropriate for the nurse educator to insist that the student change beliefs. Option D: Protecting client autonomy is included in professional nursing ethical codes, not only research ethics.

9. Answer: C

Rationale: Option A: The project should be reviewed for protection of human subjects, since it is research. Option B: The nurse educator is not required to pay students, unless that is part of the research protocol. Option C: This is the best answer since it includes approval by an institutional review board and approaches to avoid coercion. Option D: Coercion is unacceptable; thus, students must be given the option not to participate.

10. Answer: C

Rationale: Option A: The National League for Nursing provides funding and has established priorities for nursing education research; thus, C is the best answer. Option B: The National League for Nursing provides funding and has established priorities for nursing education research; thus, C is the best answer. Option C: The National League for Nursing provides funding and has established priorities for nursing education research; thus, this is the best answer. Option D: The National League for Nursing provides funding and has established priorities for nursing education research; thus, C is the best answer.

Chapter 8

1. Answer: C

Rationale: Religious seminaries are sponsored by their religious organizations to prepare clergy and laity for ministry. Academic nursing programs are found in each of the other types of institutions but not in religious seminaries.

2. Answer: D

Rationale: The academic goals of the *Future of Nursing* include preparation of 80 percent of all nurses at a baccalaureate or higher-degree level by 2020. The other options are not identified in the *Future of Nursing.*

3. Answer: A

Rationale: The traditional academic role includes a balance among teaching, scholarship, and service. The other options include activities that nurse educators may engage in, but they are not regarded as the three pillars of the academic role.

4. Answer: A

Rationale: This option best indicates respect for both the student and the faculty member and promotes civility. The other options entail action with insufficient information.

5. Answer: C

Rationale: The evidence indicates that good-quality interprofessional communication is essential for patient safety. The other options may be

outcomes, but they do not address the rationale for interprofessional education.

6. Answer: B

Rationale: The practice requirement for many nurse educators can be a particularly challenging issue for them in regard to eligibility for promotion and tenure because of the time commitment. Many academic disciplines lack a real-world practice component.

7. Answer: D

Rationale: External government regulatory bodies and accrediting agencies exercise authority over nursing programs. The other options are not evidence-based statements.

8. Answer: B

Rationale: The financial threat to academic institutions was identified as a trend that requires attention by nurse educators. The other options are not based in evidence.

9. Answer: B

Rationale: All units, including the nursing unit, need to support the institutional mission. This is expected by accrediting bodies of all nursing education programs, including those within religious institutions. The other options do not reflect professional standards.

10. Answer: C

Rationale: While academic and clinical cultures differ, professional standards require that nursing education programs promote patient safety. The other options do not reflect professional standards.

References

Billings, D. M. (2015). Culturally and linguistically responsive teaching: Part I. *The Journal of Continuing Education in Nursing, 46*(2), 62–64. doi:10.3928/00220124-20150121-14

Candela, L. (2016). Theoretical foundations of teaching and learning. In D. M. Billings & J. A. Halstead (Eds.), *Teaching in nursing: A guide for faculty* (5th ed., pp. 211–229). St. Louis, MO: Elsevier.

Caputi, L., & Frank, B. (2019). Competency I: Facilitate learning. In J. A. Halstead (Ed.), *NLN core competencies for nurse educators: A decade of influence* (pp. 17–43). Washington, DC: National League for Nursing.

Carvalho, D., Azevedo, I. C., Cruz, G. K. P., Mafra, G. A. C., Rego, A. L. C., Vitor, A.F., ... Ferreira Junior, M. A. (2017). Strategies used for the promotion of critical thinking in nursing undergraduate education: A

systematic review. *Nurse Education Today, 57,* 103–107. http://dx.doi.org/10.1016/j.nedt.2017.07.010

Efstathiou, N., & Bailey, C. (2012). Promoting active learning using Audience Response System in large bioscience classes. *Nurse Education Today, 32*(1), 91–95. doi: 10.1016/j.nedt.2011.01.017

Grossman, S. C., & Valiga, T. M. (2017). *The new leadership challenge: Creating the future of nursing* (5th ed.). Philadelphia, PA: F. A. Davis.

Lerret, S. M., & Frenn, M. (2011). Challenge with care: Reflections on teaching excellence. *Journal of Professional Nursing, 27*(6), 378–384. doi:10.1016/j.profnurs.2011.04.014

Mareno, N., Bremner, M., & Emerson, C. (2010). The use of Audience Response Systems in nursing education: Best practice guidelines. *International Journal of Nursing Education Scholarship, 7*(1), Article 32.

Retrieved from http://dx.doi.org/10.2202/1548-923X.2049

National League for Nursing (2018b). Creating community to build a civil and healthy academic work environment. *NLN Vision Series*. Retrieved from http://www.nln.org/docs/default-source/professional-development-programs/vision-statement-a-vision-for-creating-community-to-build-a-civil-and-healthy.pdf?sfvrsn=8http://www.nln.org/docs/default-source/professional-development-programs/vision-statement-a-vision-for-creating-community-to-build-a-civil-and-healthy.pdf?sfvrsn=10&pdf=VisionSeries-CreatingCommunity.

Paul, R., & Elder, L. (2013). The standards for thinking. In R. Paul & L. Elder, *Critical thinking: Tools for taking charge of your professional and personal life* (2nd ed., pp. 98–129). Upper Saddle River, NJ: Pearson Prentice Hall.

Phillips, J. M. (2016). Strategies to promote student engagement and active learning. In D. M. Billings & J. A. Halstead (Eds.), *Teaching in nursing: A guide for faculty* (5th ed., pp. 15–34). St. Louis, MO: Elsevier.

Popkess, A. M., & Frey, J. L. (2016). Strategies to support diverse learning needs of students. In D. M. Billings & J. A. Halstead (Eds.), *Teaching in nursing: A guide for faculty* (5th ed., pp. 15–34). St. Louis, MO: Elsevier, Inc.

Rasheed, S. P., Younas, A., & Sundus, A. (2018). Self-awareness in nursing: A scoping review. *Journal of Clinical Nursing, 28*, 762–774. doi: 10.1111/jocn.14708

Reader, K. J., Hamshire, C., & Chambers, A. (2017). The influence of role models in undergraduate nurse education. *Journal of Clinical Nursing, 26*, 4707–4715. doi: 10.1111/jocn.13822

Revell, S. M., & McCurry, M. K. (2010). Engaging millennial learners: Effectiveness of personal response system technology with nursing students in small and large classrooms. *Journal of Nursing Education, 49*(5), 272–275. http://dx.doi.org/10.3928/01484834-20091217-07

Rundle, S., & Dunn, R. (2008). Building excellence (BE)® BE 2000 research manual 1996–2008. Rochester, NY: Performance Concepts International.

Sedden, M. L., & Clark, K. R. (2016). Motivating students in the 21st century. *Radiologic Technology, 87*(6), 609–614.

Wiggs, C. M. (2010). Collaborative testing: Assessing teamwork and critical thinking behaviors in baccalaureate students. *Nurse Education Today, 31*(3), 279–282. doi:10.1016/j.nedt.2010.10.027.

Zaleznik, A. (1981). Managers and leaders: Are they different? *Journal of Nursing Administration, 11*(7), 25–31.

Index

Note: Page number followed by *f*, *b*, and *t* indicates figure, box, and table respectively.